THE KEY MODEL

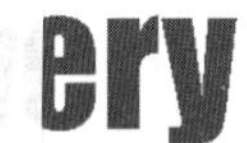

ARDAGH CLINIC

This Book is published by Ardagh Clinic
118 Stillorgan Rd,
Dublin 4,
Tel: 01-260 0118
in association with Somerville Press, Cork.

First published in Ireland October, 2004

The recommendations made in this book are generic and are not meant to replace formal medical or psychiatric diagnosis or treatment. Individuals with medical problems should always consult with their physicians about the appropriateness of following any programme and discuss appropriate modifications relevant to their unique circumstances and condition.

Not for Profit: All net profits from the sale of this book will go to fund research in applied behavioural medicine.

This book describes an innovative evidence-based programme for responding pro-actively to cancer and other serious illness. Its earlier edition, *Tipping the Scales* was published by the Ardagh Clinic in 1997

ISBN : 0-9521444-5-X
1. Cancer 2. Health 2. Psychology 3. Mind and body, 4. Holistic health

Printed in Ireland by ColourBooks Ltd
Edited by Claire Haugh
Typesetting by Kathryn O'Sullivan
Cover design, layout, and additional material: Power of 7, Ballbridge, Dublin 4.
Yoga illustrations by Hugh Collins (1977-1998)

ACKNOWLEDGEMENTS

We wish to thank:

Power of 7
Our six 'readers'
Our editor Claire Haugh
The participants in previous research groups
Deirdre Davis Brigham, who inspired us

DEDICATION

Our friend, colleague and wise mentor
Phil Walsh (died 22nd March 2004)

also Angela, Caitriona, Clare, Derrick, Geraldine,
Kevin, Louise, Mary, Michael, Olive, 'Sir' Pat,
Suzanne, the ones that got away . . .
and are still with us

FOREWORD

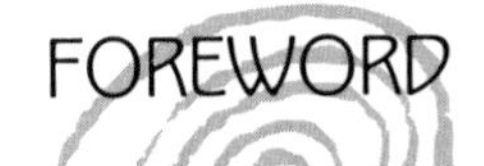

'All truth goes through three stages. First it is ridiculed. Then it is violently opposed. Finally, it is accepted as self-evident.'
SCHOEPENHOUER

Coincidentally, I was en route to the island of Crete when asked to write this foreword – just a short trip from Kos where Hippocrates (460–370 B.C.) practised his holistic medicine.

Despite being heavy tobacco growers and consumers, the Greeks have a lower risk of cardiovascular disease than other part of Europe. It has been assumed that this is due to their Mediterranean type diet. It may also be due to other lifestyle factors such as exercise, pace of life and social interaction.

The story is similar in Japan, where again in spite of heavy tobacco consumption, their Asian diet of fish, vegetables, soya products and beneficial fats, is believed to add up to low risk of disease, although apparently this is changing as a more western diet is being adopted. Researchers are currently looking at other lifestyle factors.

Recently a similar account of the Okinawa centenarians has been published. These are an island people off Japan who have adopted a traditional lifestyle. They are the oldest and healthiest authenticated group of aged people in the world. Thankfully, in addition to diet other lifestyle factors were examined, and we get a glimpse of the holistic approach that is essential for healthful living.

The cornerstone of health in my opinion is nutrition, and I agree with Hippocrates when he says, 'Let food be your medicine and medicine your food.' However, emphasising the importance of the correct fuel to heal the body is merely the starting point.

To illustrate this point I recall a story told to me by a woman whose husband was a prisoner in the World War II. They were fed similar meals for months on end – gruel and stale bread with little else. Luckily for him there was a psychologist in his group. Each day at meal times the psychologist gathered the group and they went through a different ritual of visualising the stale food as tasty nourishing chicken or meat that would replenish their depleted bodies. Interestingly, many prisoners died in other camps around them while none of his group died, and when finally released they were fitter and stronger then the men around them. This is evidence, albeit anecdotal, that the mind is a powerful place and can be used to our advantage. To quote Shakespeare, 'The mind is of its own place. It can make a heaven of hell or a hell of heaven.'

The overall message from the authors of *The Key Model*, having skilfully collated years of practice and research into an eminently readable and practical book, is that the ideas and methods outlined in the book actually work. They offer the reader, clearly and without any fuss, a means of tapping into the vast healing reserves of the mind.

I would like to compliment the authors for taking the time to forge ahead and look at new ways to help people fight back. When this book was first written (as *Tipping the Scales*, 1997), I would safely say that none of my medical colleagues had heard of psychoneuroimmunology (PNI). including myself. How things have changed in a short few years. Now the concept of PNI is much more acceptable – particularly in the area of cardiac rehabilitation where gradually more and more of these new approaches are being explored.

This book is for patients diagnosed with a life-threatening or quality-of-life threatening condition to enable them to make comprehensive, effective and well-formed choices as to their response. It draws on more than fifty years of research in psycho-behavioural medicine and twenty-five years or more in PNI from more than forty universities around the world. This new edition, *The Key Model*, also draws on the combined experience of the authors Dr. Sean Collins and Rhoda Draper in eight years of clinical research.

The authors offer us the results of solid research from universities around the world. Groundbreaking work has been done, for example, in Ohio University, where the authors of a recent review reveal that there is now sufficient data to conclude that changing psychosocial stressors can lead to actual health changes with the strongest direct evidence in infectious diseases and wound healing. Other conditions influenced are cardiovascular disease, osteoporosis, certain cancers, type2 diabetes, and frailty and functional decline. All of which confirms my belief that one should not wait for an illness to strike before engaging in the processes outlined in this book. Instead, they should be utilised as an investment in one's future good health.

This book has the potential to help you change your life if you want to. If you are a medic, do your patients a favour by drawing their attention to the book. Ireland is fortunate to have the benefits of the knowledge and expertise of these two authors who offer evidence-based methods of providing an effective adjunct to mainstream medicine and not an alternative – integrative medicine as it should be.

Having personally participated in one of the programmes outlined in the book, I was deeply impressed by the dynamism of the authors. A 'take home message' that still rings in my ears and influences daily living is 'I cannot afford the luxury of a negative thought.'

Personally I hope to be the oldest, healthiest swinger in the nursing home when the time comes!

Dr. Anne Rhatigan
MB, BCh, BAO, MICGP

CONTENTS

PART 3 – SPIRITUAL

PART 4 – THE 90-DAY PROGRAMME

PART 5 – HISTORY AND IMPORTANT CONCEPTS

PART 6 – SOME USEFUL TECHNIQUES AND INTERVENTIONS

'Lord grant me the courage to change what can be changed,
the serenity to accept what cannot be changed,
and the wisdom to know one from the other'
REINHOLD NIEBHUR (THEOLOGIAN)

INTRODUCTION

'When illness strikes suddenly, it's like unexpectedly hitting a wall at 60 mph'

'They told me I was up against a cancer survivor!' Thus commented an eminent Irish oncologist in 2001 just before going on air for a radio interview on cancer and its treatment. This is an attitude that, happily, has become less common but given the evidence, is no longer tolerable.

World statistics for cancer show that five-year survival rates vary depending on the type and the staging of the cancer. However, the overall survival rate for most cancers remain stuck at about 55%, in spite of the investment of countless millions of dollars and the work of hundreds of researchers. No significant breakthrough has so far been achieved. Any medical historian will tell you that the major reductions in disease and improvements in survival rates have come from improved housing, nutrition, hygiene, sanitation, early detection and more recently from the wonders of modern drug therapy, radiotherapy and surgery. The one remaining area for application is the influence of the mind and behaviour in cancer.

In 1990 the medical journal, *Lancet*, reported the results of a behavioural change programme which demonstrated that the progress of heart disease and, in particular, blocked arteries, could be reversed. Two years previously, another study at Stanford University in California demonstrated that the life expectancy of Stage 4 breast cancer patients could be doubled. In 1991, the Institute of Psychiatry, University of London, released the results of a 13-year study, carried out by psychologists, H.J. Eysenck and R. Grossarth-Maticek. The report showed that a particular form of psychological intervention could reduce the risk of premature death by a significant 75% among 'Type C' (cancer prone) people.

The conclusion? What a person thinks, feels, and does **can** change the odds.

Behavioural Medicine is the study of how habitual ways of thinking and acting can positively change the prospects for full recovery and more importantly how a person can be empowered to do this. Psychoneuroimmunology (PNI) is the specific study of how a person's psychological and behavioural ways can influence the immune system for the better or worse.

The principles and methods outlined in this book suggest that if a patient engages in a comprehensive and timely psychological and behavioural programme, they can significantly increase the odds of admission into the 'Winner's Circle' of those who recover from their illnesses. The 'programme' is called *The Key Model* and consists of a daily practice that includes Yoga, Meditation, Journalling, Visualisation, Breathwork etc.

Medicine has searched in vain for a single causal agent for cancer or heart disease. However, these are chronic and complex diseases. It is only when multiple elements combine together that cancer or heart disease results. Medical approaches have effectively dismissed nutrition and behaviour and ignored the mind and the spirit. However Dr Carl Simonton, co-author of the classic *Getting Well Again* commented 'There is adequate evidence that the mind potentially plays a significant role in the onset and development of cancer. Certain patterns of behaviour in response to stress contribute substantially to cancer.'

The Key Model identifies many of the co-factors (common elements) that have been shown to contribute to the development and worsening of a disease process and also more importantly, how those co-factors can be changed to improve the odds of recovery.

Although the main focus in this book is on fighting back against cancer, the same principles have been applied successfully with many other chronic conditions including: heart disease, arthritis, diabetes, asthma, fibromyalgia, as well as autoimmune diseases such as multiple sclerosis, lupus and rheumatoid arthritis.

This book has been written not as an academic textbook, but as a workbook suited to the needs of both patients and carers. With the wide availability of the Internet, further information on almost any topic described here is available at the push of a button. Academic references have therefore been kept to a minimum but are available on request. Where statements are made in the first person, these are the thoughts and opinions of both authors. Where Sean Collins is commenting, the letters (SC) follow the comment, and where Rhoda Draper is commenting, the letters (RD) follow the comment. For convenience of writing, the male gender has been used throughout.

WHAT IS NEW ABOUT THE KEY MODEL?

If there is no one single cause for cancer, it is unlikely that there will be one simple answer'
SEAN COLLINS

Numerous studies published in peer-reviewed journals from universities around the world show that genetic, physical, emotional, psychological, behavioural and spiritual aspects are all potential contributors or co-factors in cancer, yet the authors have been unable to identify a single cancer-recovery programme which comprehensively addresses all of these. The major focus continues to be on the physical body – using surgery, chemotherapy and radiotherapy.

In spite of billions of dollars in research, the overall five-year cancer survival rate has remained stuck at little more than 55%. In *The Key Model* we have attempted to identify evidence-based interventions which are currently not included in cancer recovery programmes but which may offer the potential to improve the 'survival rate' statistics. The evolving fields of psychoneuroimmunology, or PNI (how psychological and spiritual issues affect immune function) and behavioural medicine (how behaviour affects recovery) offer some exciting clues. Over a period of seven years, we have carried out pilot research programmes in Dublin exploring the effectiveness of psychological and behavioural approaches as an adjunct to conventional cancer care and seen remarkable results.

In reviewing the published literature and in pursuing long-term research, the following are specific elements which we have identified as being missing from the majority of current cancer patient recovery programmes. Each element is explored in greater detail in the book:

A programme must be **comprehensive.** This means it needs to address all of the essential elements in a patient's life: 1. Psychological and Emotional, 2. Physical, Behavioural and Nutritional, 3. Spiritual, and 4. The role of Chaos or Luck. Up until now, behavioural medicine interventions have tended to be offered on an 'a la Carte' basis with the patient 'cherry picking' elements that took his fancy, only to produce wildly varying and often disappointing results.

An effective recovery programme needs a detailed review of the patient's life for the presence of evidence-based negative co-factors which may have contributed to the development of the disease and which, when removed or corrected, can contribute to full recovery.

Programmes need a similar review of the patient's life to identify evidence-based positive co-factors, the absence of which may have led to the development of the condition and which, if introduced now, may contribute to full recovery.

Provided time is available, psychological, behavioural and nutritional approaches are best introduced before the patient has received conventional treatment. Research suggests that such approaches can often improve the patient's capacity to derive best benefit from the treatment. They also have been shown to enhance the effectiveness of the treatment. A **timely** introducing of these elements is crucial.

Behavioural medicine programmes must insist on sustained application of individual interventions until the critical mass point (as identified in research) is reached.

Patients often know 'what' they could be doing to help themselves towards recovery. However, they often find themselves lacking the 'how' – the skill or the motivation to do it. Behavioural medicine programmes need to provide patients with the specific tools and skills for psychological, behavioural and nutritional change. They must also leave the patient with a sense of personal empowerment rather than a sense of dependence.

It is essential that patients are provided with an awareness of the potential for inadvertent hindering by certain medical personnel, and with the tools to counter this.

The placebo effect is a proven powerful phenomenon and needs to be viewed as an asset to be harnessed rather than as a nuisance to be factored out.

Appropriate levels of challenge (a fundamental requirement) in the realms of the physical, emotional/psychological and the spiritual should be provided.

The concept of the patient and medical team together crafting an 'Optimum Environment' in which automated self-healing can occur needs to be pursued.

The Key Model looks to address all of these factors
in a 90-day programme. (*See* page 115)

THE SIGNIFICANCE OF CO-FACTORS IN RECOVERY

Some years ago, I (SC) was a 'keynote' speaker at a professional conference on psychological approaches to serious illness. The audience of academics and scientists were committed to answering the question: 'What is the single significant element in any treatment programme that makes the difference between responding well to medical treatment or poorly?'

My opening statement was, 'I'm a keynote speaker and this is my key' at the same time holding up my front door key. I then posed the question, 'As scientists, will any member of this learned audience tell me which is the "significant" serration or notch on this key?' Silence followed. The answer of course is that no single one is significant. Each individual notch is important and, furthermore, a raised section on my key may well be a indented section on someone else's.

Human beings are unique and complex, far more so than a front door key. Why then do we believe there is a single solution or treatment that will suit all patients? A recent study showed that when healthy people are exposed to the cold virus, placed directly on the mucous membrane of the nose, only approximately 12% of subjects developed a cold. I ask myself 'Why?'

When scientists design experiments, they try to have only one variable element present, and stabilise all other factors. This requires the deletion of a 'complex dynamic environment'. It works well in the laboratory but it ignores the complexity of each unique individual.

In our comprehensive searching, we found that researchers have identified more than one hundred co-factors which have shown to potentially contribute to the onset and progression of chronic diseases such as cancer. These researchers also identified more than twenty psychological and behavioural interventions that have been shown to measurably contribute to recovery and spontaneous remission among patients. Will any of these interventions cure a particular illness? The answer is 'Probably not.' Can they contribute to a measurable recovery, particularly when used in combination? The answer is, 'Yes!' And that is what this book is about.

A major problem in exploring psychological and behavioural interventions is that researchers tend to explore just one or two elements at a time. This approach is like trying it use flour alone to bake bread. It is the complex co-mingling and interaction of the various ingredients (water, yeast, flour, heat etc.) that produces good bread. Therefore we suggest that many behavioural medicine programmes are potentially flawed in that they include only a limited number of approaches in a haphazard fashion. Although they occasionally show some positive effects, they often fail for the simple reason that they are not comprehensive or sustained.

Now let's look at medicine and its approach to the treatment of disease. Currently virtually all attention is on treating the physical body, the disease and the symptoms. Little attention is given to the person, the mind and the emotions. Even less attention is given to changing unhealthy behaviours or healing emotional trauma, inspite of strong evidence that these are often significant factors to the onset and progression of a disease such as cancer.

Dr Hans Selye, the undisputed 'father' of modern stress research suggested: 'Our experiments and studies of multi-causal diseases have taught us that many maladies are the result of a constellation of factors amongst which non-specific stress often plays a decisive role.' He made this comment almost 50 years ago!

It is worth wondering, if cancer is 100% physical, environmental or genetic in origin, why don't animals develop cancers in the same proportions or with the same frequency as we do? The human ability to self-observe is the major factor that makes us different from animals. Could it be that the psychological or 'self observation' aspect in humans is the important additive factor?

Daniel Goleman, author of *Emotional Intelligence*, commented, 'People who experience chronic anxiety, long periods of sadness and pessimism, unremitting tension or incessant hostility, relentless cynicism or suspiciousness have double the risk of diseases such as asthma, arthritis, headaches, peptic ulcers and heart disease. This makes these emotions comparable to smoking or high cholesterol in terms of being a risk factor.'

Patients all too frequently are tempted to leave the responsibility to the doctors. However if your house was on fire and you had a lunch engagement, would you go to lunch and leave it all to the firemen? Of course you wouldn't! Yet many patients still 'leave it all' to the doctors. The behavioural medicine programme described here offers a viable evidence-based approach.

~ SUMMARY ~

Cancer is a complex disease with has no identified single cause.

It is unlikely to have one single solution!

PART 1

PSYCHOLOGICAL AND EMOTIONAL

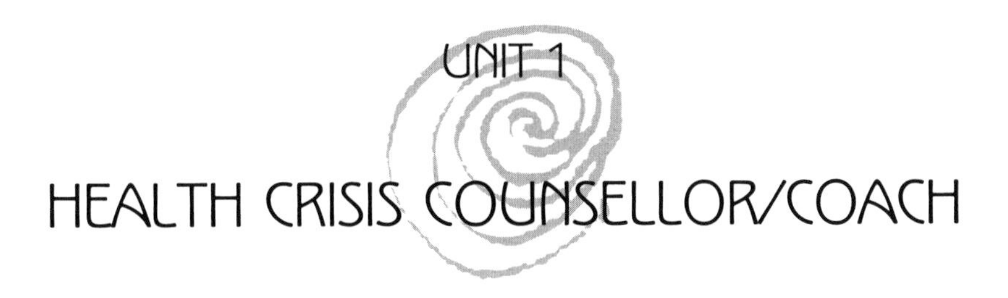

UNIT 1

HEALTH CRISIS COUNSELLOR/COACH

'Give sorrow words: the grief that does not speak,
Whispers the o'er-fraught heart and bids it break'
WILLIAM SHAKESPEARE

If you're dealing with a major health problem, you're likely to have been catapulted onto an emotional rollercoaster without warning. You may know 'what' you could be doing in order to be healthier, but still having trouble coming up the 'how' to carry it out.

Research suggests that having a clear-headed person fill the role of crisis counsellor/coach, results in: a) a greater effectiveness in designing a fight-back plan and, b) a far greater probability of sticking to that plan. In an ideal situation, you would call on a professional specifically trained for this role. In reality, however, the task generally falls on caring, but untrained, shoulders.

The following are some simple guidelines to help you in identifying a person or persons who might fill that role, and to guide that person in knowing how best to help you.

SOME POTENTIAL MENTORS/COUNSELLORS

- Professional health-crisis counsellor (*See* Appendix 3 page 211)
- Specialist nurse/counsellor (trained for your disease/condition)
- GP, doctor or nurse (may be too busy or may require specific training)
- General counsellor/psychologist/psychotherapist (may require specific skills and knowledge)
- Family member
- Close friend
- Relative
- Work colleague

THE ROLE OF A HEALTH CRISIS COUNSELLOR

Counselling refers to a 'helping' process, the aim of which is not to change someone, but to help him access resources he already has to enable him to cope or adapt effectively.

GUIDELINES FOR EFFECTIVE COUNSELLING

- The sharing of worries or concerns in a confidential environment.
- Be in a 'therapeutic' relationship, i.e. the counsellor gives up his own thoughts and interests and gives complete attention to the patient. It has been defined as: 'taking responsibility for having someone else experience feeling understood by you'.
- Facilitate and encourage the patient towards self-help.
- Look to open up choices and options for them.
- Look to understand the practical and psychological problems of living with a serious illness, and help to develop specific skills to address these.
- Facilitate the patient to stay on track through regular review sessions.
- Help the person when he 'falls off the horse', or becomes disheartened (particularly during treatment).

FEATURES OF A 'THERAPEUTIC' RELATIONSHIP

- Concreteness – Accurately assisting in identifying the problem and defining a well-formed outcome.
- Time-scale – Addressing, from the outset, the actual time needed for implementing a programme for recovery, and to modify this as the process evolves (for patient and mentor). Just as disease takes time to develop, recovery too is a progression and takes time.
- Confrontation – Addressing essential and material issues honestly where appropriate. This does not imply aggressiveness. It means constructively pointing out discrepancies between the patient's intentions and what he actually does!
- Increased awareness – Encouraging the patient towards increased self-understanding.
- Understanding/Empathy/Warmth – Ensuring that the patient feels, without reservation, that he is understood, accepted and responded to genuinely by his counsellor/coach.

- Expressiveness – Encouraging the patient towards honest disclosure, and to becoming assertive and immediate in his reactions and responses.
- Open communication – Openness from the counsellor and, when necessary, confronting the patient but without playing the role of advisor or helper.

IN A COUNSELLING ROLE

Don't . . .

Interrupt – Panic or look anxious – Interpret
Misinterpret – Look out the window – Judge and evaluate
Direct and lead more than is necessary – Take responsibility for change
Blame, moralise, preach or patronise – Label or diagnose
Make judgements – Humour just to have the client feel good
Advise and/or teach (You 'should' or 'ought') – Interrogate
Over-interpret – Talk about yourself excessively or inappropriately
Automatically compare the patient's experience with your own
Try to put on a professional facade – Fake attention
Force the patient to be too brief – Have an answer for everything
Minimise or discount the client's feelings about what he sees as a major trauma
Invalidate the patient's feelings.

IN A COUNSELLING ROLE

Do . . .

Help find out what problems there are
Help in developing a well-formed outcome
Help to identify and access resources
Challenge where appropriate
Communicate energy and commitment
Be an attentive listener
Remember to 'shut up' sometimes
Be kind to yourself

~ SUMMARY ~

*When you have a health crisis counsellor/coach,
you are more likely to feel supported, deal effectively
with challenges and stay on track.*

UNIT 2

DEVELOPING A WELL-FORMED OUTCOME

The unconscious mind, which effectively manages your body on a moment-to-moment basis, is best guided or motivated by a precise, well-defined outcome. The pilot on a 767 leaving Heathrow for New York will program into his auto pilot the exact co-ordinates for his destination. Why would you be any different?

Goals, or clear objectives, cause you to focus attention. They cause you to prioritise how you use your energy and resources. A patient confronting serious illness often experiences confusion in his thinking and fails to specify exactly what he wants to achieve. Instead he will often focus on what he doesn't want.

The following brief model for developing a Well-Formed Outcome (WFO) is used with excellent results in such diverse areas as medicine, business and counselling. There is an old saying: 'If you fail to plan . . . you plan to fail!' Take the time to find as many answers as possible to the following questions in order to enhance the clarity and effectiveness of your unconscious thinking. This exercise is best done in writing.

ANSWER AS FULLY AS YOU CAN

- What is your outcome? What specifically do you want to have happen (rather than what you don't want to happen!).
- What specifically are you already doing to achieve that outcome, and what stage are you at now in terms of achieving this?
- What new things can you, and will you, be doing in the future to ensure achieving that outcome?
- What, specifically, will achieving that outcome do for YOU? How will you benefit?
  - In the short-term?
  - In the long-term?
- Who else will benefit? (partner, family, work-colleagues, etc.)
- How, specifically, will they benefit?
- Is the outcome just for you? For others? What others? Why for them?

- How specifically will you know when you've achieved your outcome? What evidence will you need to know that you have achieved your objective?
- What stops you now, or might stop you in the future?
- What specific additional resources, information, skills etc. do you, or might you, need to put in place?
- When do you need to have these resources in place?
- What will you gain from achieving your outcome?
- What will happen if you succeed?
- What will happen if you don't succeed?
- What, if anything, will you lose by achieving your outcome?
- Is achieving your outcome worthwhile? Summarise for yourself why!

~ SUMMARY ~

When you develop a Well-Formed Outcome,
you programme your unconscious mind for automated
self-healing and recovery.

KEY NOTES

'The interventions are scientific, rational and practical. With a little organisation I incorporated them into my working day. I found the philosophy of the programme very good. Attending alone gave me a lift.' *L.M., Dundalk*

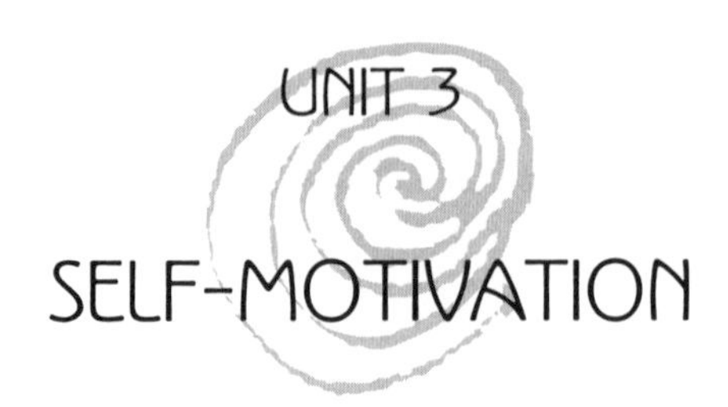

UNIT 3
SELF-MOTIVATION

The road to hell, they say, is paved with good intentions! How often have you said, 'I'm going to try and get up early and take a brisk walk.' or 'I'm going to try to avoid eating biscuits.' Maybe you are a rare paragon of virtue in these matters, however most of us can identify with having had similar good intentions but, when tempted by a warm bed or a steaming mug of coffee and a slice of cake, give in. Words such as: 'I deserve it!' come to mind. We often hear smokers say, 'It's the only pleasure I have in life!'

The problem with motivation is that it is often driven by short-term goals, such as that lie-in, that coffee, that cake, that cigarette. We seldom look to the future – imagining how life will be for us when we have managed to take that healthy walk, to avoid junk food and to stay free of cigarettes. Most of us tend to procrastinate especially when we are relatively healthy. We feel that we will 'get around to' a healthier lifestyle one of these days. The fact that we might begin to feel better, look better and have more energy is seldom a powerful motivator for us. However, if you are a health-challenged person you do not have time on your side. Now is the only time to start.

The secret to self-motivation lies in your ability to 'visualise' how life will change when you no longer have the disease; and using your 'mind's eye' to see yourself doing what needs to be done. Before you go to bed, 'see yourself' getting up at the time you plan to get up. See yourself shopping for the foods that will be healthy and nourishing. See yourself successfully engaging in all the individual aspects of your health programme. Set mini-goals, and see yourself achieving them. Visualise the results, 'vividly and in detail', and your powerful unconscious mind will keep you on target.

Self-motivation is also considerably easier when you are pursuing an objective, such as optimum health, as part of a group under the guidance of a skilled and passionate facilitator.

~ SUMMARY ~

The word 'motivation' has the same origins as the word emotion. If you can trigger strong positive emotion around your outcome, you are more likely to succeed.

KEY NOTES

'I would say that reading the book and doing the programme was the biggest life-changing experience I had . . . . It taught me how to make choices to benefit my day-to-day living and gave me new energy for life.' *A.H., Wexford*

UNIT 4

ELIMINATING DISTRACTIONS AND 'VAMPIRES'

The 'vampires' are the heralds of doom – those 'helpful' friends who insist on telling you the worst; media people who publish misinformation in headlines to grab your attention; healthcare professionals who don't believe in your potential to recover. These people can drain your energy and need to be ruthlessly purged from your life if you are seriously engaged in a fight-back programme. Beliefs can heal but also can kill. What you read, what you watch on TV, who you spend time with, what you focus on – they have all been shown to impact on your immune system and your healing prospects. I (SC) remember a patient reporting a sense that his family had become weary of the illness and the treatments and wished he would either recover or die, but please 'stop this hanging about in the middle!'

About ten years ago, a woman came to see me (SC) with a strange story and carrying two medical folders and a cardboard box. She had been diagnosed two and a half years previously with an untreatable advanced cancer. The first file contained her medical notes confirming the pathology and the negative prognosis. She had been given just twelve to eighteen months to live. She embarked on a journey that took her to a medical doctor in the US who worked in an unconventional way with so-called 'hopeless cases'. She spent three months attending this doctor and, lo and behold, her cancer went into complete remission and she regained full health. The second file contained her revised diagnosis and positive prognosis.

She came to see me because she felt confused. The box she had brought along contained a 'device' supplied to her by the doctor in the US. This 'device', to say the least, was bizarre. It comprised of a large crystal bound in copper wire, a light source and various wires and electrodes that could be attached to the body. She spent time every day attached to this device. I could not think of any mechanism by which this device could have had any possible effect on her pathology – yet the evidence was there in her medical files!

She described her confusion as follows: Although she had achieved a proven remission, it was only recently she had begun to tell her friends of her daily ritual with this strange device. Many of her friends told her that she was 'out of her mind', that such a ridiculous device could not possibly be of any benefit. She had now become uncertain as to whether or not she was fooling herself by using it. My advice to her was to keep doing what obviously had been working for her. Six months later I read of her death. When I spoke to her son, he told me of his mother's eventual abandonment of this ritual with the device along with her subsequent loss of belief in her 'cure' and loss of hope for her future.

My own feelings on this case were that perhaps she had somehow managed to harness the much spoken-of powers of the placebo response (*See* page 178) – the magical combination of the powers of belief and expectation – along with the mysterious and sometimes elusive self-healing mechanisms of the human body. I still wonder if her 'friends' had served her well?

~ SUMMARY ~

Clear all negative people and situations out of your life.
They can kill you!

KEY NOTES

'The programme taught me the practice of new strategies and skills to deal with day-to-day managements of my thinking and emotions, . . . The feeling of support and compassion was very helpful and healing within the group.' *V.H., Co. Laois*

UNIT 5

CHANGING UNHELPFUL BELIEFS, ATTITUDES AND MIND-SETS

Your beliefs determine your response or sense of power in relation to everyday events. As a patient, some of these beliefs will be empowering, such as, 'I have a powerful self-healing body'. Some may be negative or disempowering, such as, 'I'm never going to get well'. Negative beliefs can deny a person access to their own capabilities and de-motivate them.

To quote Henry Ford, 'Whether you believe you can, or whether you believe you can't, you're right!' Most of our beliefs are simple generalisations from the past, based on our interpretations of both painful and pleasurable experiences. Our beliefs, however, do have a significant impact on our ability to think, to do things and, most importantly, to motivate ourselves. Beliefs are, however, nothing more than a sense of certainty about something.

Beliefs do not just bring about psychological change. They also cause physical changes in the body. If you are caught doing something you believe to be wrong, how long does it take to blush? In the context of healing, beliefs are neither right nor wrong. What is important is whether they are they helpful. If a person believes himself to have an incurable and fatal disease, what is the likelihood of a cure?

HOW TO CHALLENGE UNHELPFUL BELIEFS

Step 1: Make a list of any 'disempowering' or limiting beliefs which you currently hold about yourself, your body, your health or your prognosis. Include any negative belief in your ability to motivate yourself to do what needs to be done to create an opportunity for optimum recovery.

Step 2: Make a list of potentially 'empowering' or useful beliefs which you currently hold about yourself, your body, your healing capability and your ability to motivate yourself. (Remember that most beliefs were useful at one time or in some particular context. However, this usefulness can, and often does, change with the passage of time.)

Step 3: Now begin to challenge the limiting or disempowering beliefs, one at a time.

- How is this belief ridiculous or absurd?
- Where, or from whom, did I get this belief? Is there an alternative?
- Was this a worthwhile source?
- What will it ultimately cost me emotionally if I don't let go of this belief?
- What will it ultimately cost me health-wise if I don't let go of this belief?
- What will it ultimately cost me in relationships if I don't let go of this belief?
- How specifically will my life change for the better when I have dumped this belief?
- What belief(s) would be more useful? Who currently has belief(s) like this? What can I do to acquire such belief(s)?
- What is the longest time a person has survived (with quality of life) with this condition/disease? What did they do? Ask your doctor!

Consider repeating this challenge, in writing, for four to five days. Use self-hypnosis (*See* page 34) to replace any unhelpful beliefs or to install any new belief(s)!

~ SUMMARY ~

Your beliefs are not cast in stone. If they are potential blocks to recovery, you can change them using this process.

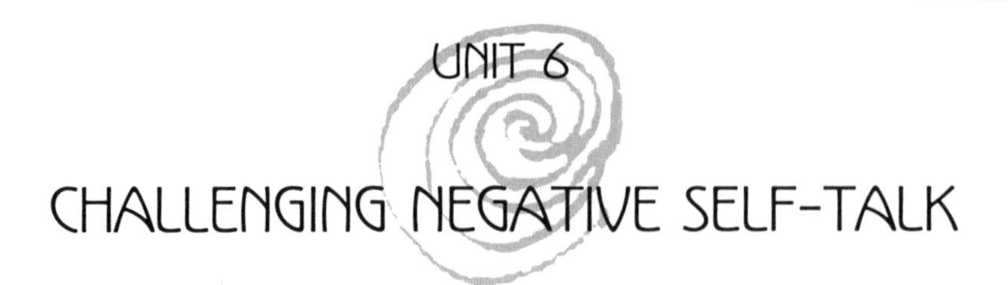

UNIT 6

CHALLENGING NEGATIVE SELF-TALK

'Fear makes come true what one is afraid of.'
VICTOR FRANKL

It's not what happens to us in life that is important; rather, it's the way we respond to those events that counts. The habitual questions we ask ourselves such as, 'Why does this always happen to me?' or 'Why are other people so lucky?' will determine the way we interpret and evaluate our day-to-day experiences, and ultimately the quality of our lives.

When serious illness strikes, a patient's internal conversation becomes even more important. Whatever a person focusses on tends to expand. Depression, which has a suppressing effect on the immune system, is frequently triggered by rumination and negative internal conversations – in other words, what a person is focusing on. Psychologist Dr. Albert Ellis, developer of 'Rational Emotive Behavioural Therapy' called this practice 'Awfulising'. Of course, it would be unfair to deny that a diagnosis of life-threatening illness is 'awful'. However, we must be vigilant in distinguishing between what is fact and what is not. Alfred Adler said, 'It is very obvious that we are not influenced by "facts" but by our interpretation of the facts.'

Researchers and writers, such as Dr. Tom Rusk, Anthony Robbins and Steve Andreas, Ph.D., encourage us to ask ourselves 'different' questions from those we usually ask, so as to shift 'habitual' orientation! 'What am I happy about?' or 'What was one pleasant experience I had today?'

SEVEN-DAY CHALLENGE

For a period of seven days, explore starting each morning by asking yourself the following specific questions and really committing to exploring the answers that emerge. Of course it's easier to ask yourself the other 'awfulising' questions – but is it useful?

In my life right now . . .

- What am I happy about?
- What *could* I be happy about? (Go on . . . find some things!)
- What am I excited about?
- What *could* I be excited about?
- What am I proud of?
- What *could* I be proud of?
- What am I grateful for?
- What else *could* I be grateful for?
- What do I really enjoy in life and how often am I doing it?
- What am I committed to?
- What *could* I be committed to?
- Who do I love and who loves me?
- What could I actively do, *today*, to improve any, or all, of those relationships?
- With any event or occurrence that went 'poorly' yesterday, what positive thing could I have learned from that experience that would allow me to let go of any negative feelings and feel happier?
- Make sure to write down your responses to the above questions as this can make them more meaningful.

~ SUMMARY ~

Negative emotions suppress the immune system and recovery. Positive emotions make recovery more probable. Negative self-talk is just a habit – and it takes just three weeks to change that habit!

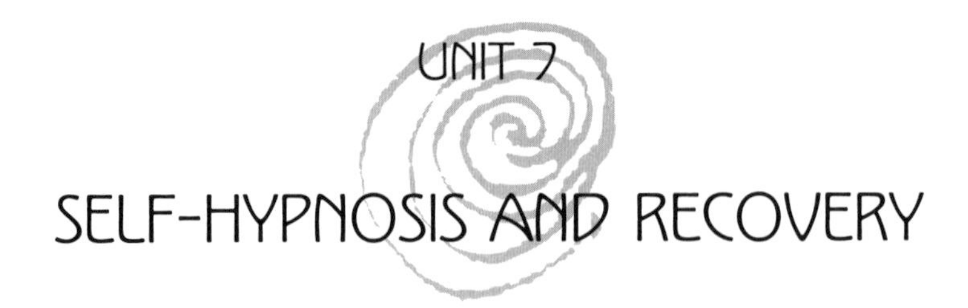

UNIT 7

SELF-HYPNOSIS AND RECOVERY

Many people have mystical views about hypnosis – an area of specialisation of ours for over 27 years (between us). At one time, hypnosis lay outside medical practice, but since the 1940s it has become an established and approved area of mainstream medicine throughout the world.

HYPNOSIS

Fundamental elements of hypnosis are belief and expectation. Hypnosis is defined as an altered state of awareness in which the unconscious mind is open to suggestion, suggestion that may well be the opposite of what was previously believed. When you are trying to recover from an illness, you are particularly susceptible to inadvertent hypnosis from yourself and others (*See* Voodoo Death, page 158). As well as diagnosis and treatment, belief and expectation are what the medical profession offer. Your choice is to determine whether their belief and expectation will be positive or negative!

THE MIND

In Freud's early model of the mind, he described it as being like an iceberg floating in the ocean, the small area above the water equating to the 'conscious' or 'thinking' part of the mind and the vast area beneath the water equating to the 'unconscious'. Although he later modified this theory somewhat, for the purpose of simplicity in this text, you can consider your 'unconscious' to be everything outside of your normal consciousness or awareness.

THE UNCONSCIOUS

The unconscious is like a vast 'reference library' in which you store every event, emotion and feeling from the moment of your birth to the present moment. Also in here are stored all of the automated reactions and responses you use to enable you to deal with everyday life. Surgeon Wilder Penfield won a Nobel Prize in 1969 for demonstrating that everything we have experienced is stored in the unconscious. Therefore, your reaction to any new experience will be substantially influenced, or perhaps even dictated, by what you have experienced in the past.

Whenever you find yourself challenged in any way, the 'researcher' in your unconscious mind scans the relevant files stored in its vast 'library'. Then, based on your previous experiences, beliefs and values, your mind delivers back a way of responding to that situation. The answer that comes instantaneously is a brief, generalised answer, rather than a stream of previous, similar experiences. The mind sifts through, deletes, distorts and generalises virtually all incoming information, allowing the conscious mind to get on with the tasks in hand. This demonstrates to us what a fast, powerful computer we have at our disposal.

Whenever your conscious mind encounters a request for information, 'researchers' scan the files stored in the 'library' of your unconscious. Then, combined with your beliefs and values, your mind delivers to you a way of responding or reacting to a given situation. The response delivered is not a digital stream of previous similar experiences but is a generalised, abbreviated, instantaneous 'answer'.

THE CRITICAL FACTOR

An important part of the mind is to act as 'critic'. It is the mind that evaluates all incoming information and selects which beliefs, ideas, concepts, etc. are accepted into the unconscious 'library'. Equally important, it is the mind that decides which ones are to be rejected. For instance, a person who overhears a suggestion that 'the world is flat' might soon find himself the subject of some derision if his mind decides to accept rather than reject that idea?

In the context of clinical hypnotherapy, we are encouraging you to introduce to your mind some new and more useful suggestions, behaviour or habitual ways of thinking. However, these new ways may be at variance with the 'status quo' in your unconscious 'library'. The 'workers ' in your 'library' might be holding on firmly to the belief: 'I am an anxious person and that's how I am – full stop!' In this instance, the critical factor (the mind) is an unwitting block to positive progress. In order to install an alternative program or more useful belief system, it is necessary to bypass this critical part of your mind, and this where hypnosis and self-hypnosis prove useful.

PROGRAMMING

The formula or recipe used for 'programming' or changing the unconscious mind is as follows:

- Accepting Personal Responsibility for Change (AR) – Desirable
- A Relaxed Body (RB) – Desirable
- Relaxed Mind with Imagination (RM) – Desirable
- Strong Emotion (SE) – Essential
- Suggestion (SG) – Essential

When combined in this sequence = Powerful Programming

The Laws of Suggestion say that if you receive a suggestion at the same time as you are experiencing a strong emotion (either positive or negative), it is likely to be accepted without normal critical evaluation. A person who has just received a diagnosis of a life-threatening or 'quality-of-life'-threatening disease is highly susceptible to suggestion from physicians, family and friends alike. Professor Herbert Benson: 'The naming of an illness usually installs new and generally negative messages in the brain'

Suggestions are often accepted like a 'hex' and frequently make matters worse. The timing of a suggestion in relation to the experiencing of a strong emotion is critical. If the suggestion is made or imagined just before, or at the peak of, the strong emotion, a dramatically increased programmed response is created. If the suggestion is made after the peak of the emotional response, the programming effect will likely be minimal. The manner in which a doctor communicates a diagnosis and prognosis is therefore crucial. If you feel that your mind has accepted a harmful suggestion, it is very important that you clear it from your mind, perhaps with the help of a therapist.

INTENSITY OF EMOTION

The strength or impact of programming is in direct proportion to the intensity of emotion experienced simultaneous with suggestion – the stronger the emotion, the stronger the programming.

REPETITION

Where a low intensity of emotion is experienced, repetition or continuous exposure can compensate and still result in unwanted programming. Television advertising is an example of this repetitive exposure or patterning.

IMAGINATION

Having been severely stung as a child, I (SC) have a strong dislike of wasps. However, I find honeybees interesting, harmless creatures – if I treat them with respect. Last summer, a little flying creature came buzzing into my office. Instantly, I got a cold shiver and the hair stood up on my arms. It was only a bumblebee – but my imagination, belief and expectation had triggered an instantaneous response in my body. Most of you will have had similar experiences.

PHOBIAS AS AN EXAMPLE OF CONDITIONING

In psychology, phobias provide us with a wonderful example of the principles of hypnotic conditioning in action. The following is an actual case with some details changed to protect confidentiality.

> A female client, Mary, was flying from London Heathrow to Malta on a surprise one-week winter holiday with her husband.
>
> Before her marriage, she had flown many times over a good number of years as an executive secretary with her employer. Flying was a familiar and comfortable experience for her.
>
> The children and pets had been safely left with the grandparents.
>
> It was a cold January back home, and Mary and her husband were looking forward to enjoying a lazy week in the sun. She was now in a relaxed state (RB) sitting on the plane, forty minutes out of Heathrow. Her mind was relaxed, perhaps imagining herself (RM), sitting on the beach or by the pool, soaking up the warm sun and sipping a cool drink.
>
> Suddenly, the plane hits an air-pocket and drops abruptly. Coffee spills, lights flash, the aircraft frame groans, people scream and Mary experiences a strong emotion (SE), terror!
>
> Nearing the peak of this strong emotion, in her mind she says to herself something like, 'The plane's going to crash, we're all going to die' and simultaneously, creates or recalls pictures in her mind of previous aircraft disasters she may have seen on television or in the papers (SG).

Soon the plane levels out, the coffee is mopped up and things are back to normal . . . or are they? In her conscious mind, Mary knows that flying is safe. She consciously knows this – because she's sitting in a plane! However, she has just gone through all the necessary steps for powerful self-hypnotic conditioning: (RB + RM + SE + SG = Powerful Programming or Conditioning).

Into her subconscious mind, without any 'critical judgement', has crept a suggestion or new belief. Even though her actual suggestion was, 'The plane's going to crash, we're all going to die!' her mind will likely generalise this into, 'All planes crash!' She now experiences major conflict in her mind, on one hand her conscious mind is saying, 'Flying is safe' and, on the other hand, the unconscious is saying, 'All planes crash!'

Whenever such conflict exists, the subconscious will always win, as it's a presupposition that everything in the unconscious is 'true'. Such information in theory has already gone through critical evaluation or 'quality control'. Without this presupposition, a person would be unable to 'know' how to interact with his/her environment because they could not rely on the 'reference library'.

Mary returned from her holiday by boat and train and was unwilling to fly until she came for therapy in 1991. Her phobic response was successfully resolved within three sessions of hypnotherapy.

THE WONDER OF PHOBIC CONDITIONING

When a person develops an unhelpful belief system, it may well last for life if left unresolved.

In the above example, it only took Mary a matter of seconds to install this life-long belief system.

The programming of her unconscious mind was based on a synthetic experience. In other words: the plane never crashed nor did anyone die. Mary simply imagined the threat to her life, vividly and in detail. Dr. Maxwell Maltz reminds us that: 'The subconscious mind cannot differentiate between a real experience and one imagined vividly and in detail.'

1. Phobic responses do occasionally diminish over time, generally due to what is called systematic desensitisation – regular, but distanced, exposure to the feared object or situation.

2. This type of negative programming may lie sleeping in the unconscious for years before causing problems. Frequently people will have no conscious memory of the original event, yet they can find themselves behaving or reacting irrationally, or in a way that is not in agreement with their conscious belief system. At one level of mind, they know that what they are thinking and feeling is crazy and uncalled-for yet, at another level, they believe wholeheartedly in the irrational belief . . . what a mess!

Dr Ernest Rossi reports a 1995 study by Ruzyla-Smith showing that hypnosis can deliver a measurable increase in immune function as measured by B-cells and helper T-cells. It offers, therefore, a potent and useful tool.

BEHAVIOURAL CHANGE PRINCIPLES AND HYPNOSIS

Eeffective remission or cure tends to come from a combination of the best of modern medicine along with a radical change in lifestyle. Most people know 'what' they should be doing, in terms of exercise, diet, quiting smoking, and thinking, but find it very difficult to actually know 'how' to deliver the goods. Old habits and patterns get in the way.

Also, when people are challenged or upset, they frequently resort to many of their least healthy behaviours – overeating, drinking and smoking – as a means of finding comfort, even though this is the opposite of what they know they should be doing. This is where psychological interventions such as counselling, hypnotherapy or NLP (Neuro-Linguistic Programming) can be helpful. Learning to develop skills with self-hypnosis and visualisation are effective ways for a person to break through old habits and patterns.

It is essential that a 'fight-back' programme should include a review of such behaviour and thinking patterns, as well as a specific and timely strategy for resolving them. If this is not done at an early stage, future efforts will be constantly undermined. Paradoxically, overcoming old unwanted habits is often easier when we are ill, and this tends to bring about a sense of pride and accomplishment that supports a 'taking charge' mind-set.

When catastrophe strikes, it often frustrates the patient's major hopes, dreams and ambitions. Patients frequently squander scarce mental and physical energy trying to continue to pursue these hopes and dreams. A critical aspect in behavioural medicine is to examine coping styles or coping ability. Those who respond with despair often die prematurely. Those who respond with the perception of a 'challenge' will likely thrive (*See* Characteristics of the Miracle Prone, page 170). Studies show that such a mind-set (referred to as 'internal locus of control') leads to improved immune function, faster recovery and better overall health.

Studies of survivors of concentration camps in World War II showed a common attitude was the implicit belief that their destiny lay in their own hands. They rarely, if ever, doubted that their own resources would be sufficient to allow them to determine their fate. Most patients are capable of developing such a helpful mind-set using self-hypnosis.

EMPOWERING MEDICATION

In relation to medical treatment, we have found that patients can use hypnosis or self-hypnosis to enhance the effectiveness of existing drugs. This allows them to reduce the inevitable stress-loading on the body and the side-effects of the medication. Hypnosis has a long history in the effective management of pain and the treatment of side effects.

INSTRUCTIONS FOR LEARNING SELF-HYPNOSIS OR SELF-PROGRAMMING

1. Find somewhere quiet and comfortable where you won't be disturbed.
2. Sit in a comfortable chair for a few moments and gently become aware of your breathing.
3. Pick a spot to focus on, just above your line of vision (without tilting the head). Allow the eyes to stay focussed on this spot for about two minutes without moving your gaze.
4. Keeping your eyes elevated, allow your eyelids to close gently.
5. As your eyelids close down, immediately take a long deep breath . . . and then . . . exhale slowly . . . and as you do so, imagine the sensation of floating . . . (in the sea, in the bath, wherever) . . . and as you feel that sensation, and keeping one elbow on the arm of the chair, begin to float your dominant hand slowly upwards into a vertical position.
6. As you float your hand upward, repeat to yourself (in your mind), 'My hand is floating up, my hand is floating up, my hand is floating . . .', without interruption, until your hand is vertical. (The purpose of this repetition is to keep the conscious mind occupied!)
7. As soon as the hand is upright, offer an appropriate suggestion to yourself. Self-suggestions or programming should be stated positively (what you want rather than what you don't want.)

Repeat your suggestion twice, allowing time for assimilation and, where possible, visualising or imagining the positive results. Your objective is to make the goal attractive to the unconscious mind.

(Work on only one suggestion per session. Prepare, and write down or memorise, your suggestion in advance! You may also open your eyes briefly to read your suggestion.)

8. When you've completed the suggestion or visualisation, immediately return your mind back to the floating sensation in your hand and now, start repeating to yourself (without interruption), 'My hand is floating down, my hand is floating down, my hand is floating down . . .'
9. When your hand has returned to a relaxed position, open your eyes and allow yourself a few moments to re-orient. You are building a new mental muscle!!!

(Modified from the work of Dr David Spiegel)

SUGGESTED TIMES

1. When you wake up
2. Before you leave for school or work
3. At lunch-time
4. On returning from school or work
5. Before going to sleep.

Note: To learn the self-hypnosis technique correctly, it needs to be practiced at least 5 to 6 times a day for 14 consecutive days. These training sessions take about two minutes from start to finish and should be enjoyable.

(*Trance and Treatment* by Professor David Spiegel and Dr Herbert Spiegel, 1978.)

~ SUMMARY ~

You cannot 'not' practice self-hypnosis, You can choose to do it purposefully, intentionally and for your own benefit.

SAMPLE SUGGESTIONS FOR SELF-HYPNOSIS

Cancer:	'My immune function is strengthening by 10% each day' 'The cancer cells are weakening with each passing day' 'The chemotherapy/radiation therapy is accurately targeting and destroying the cancer cells successfully' 'The tumour is shrinking by 15% each day and will soon be gone'
Energy:	'As I now care for my body and give it rest, my energy increases by 10% each day. I accept that there will be days when my body will want more rest and this is OK'
Stress:	'I am becoming more calm and relaxed with each passing day' 'I now have the ability to push my 'pause' button when I feel myself becoming stressed'
Pain:	'Pain is an important messenger. However, the discomfort I have been feeling is no longer necessary, and is decreasing by 20% every day.'
Nausea:	'The treatment I'm receiving is highly effective. As I develop my ability to be calm and relaxed, the side-effects are going away'
Sleep:	'As I develop my ability to relax each day, I now fall into a deep and peaceful sleep within a short time of lying down to rest' 'When I complete this self-hypnosis session, I will fall into a deep and restful sleep'
Fear:	'My confidence in my body, its ability to heal and to make the best use of my treatment, grows with each passing day'
Medication:	'The tablets/treatment I'm taking become(s) stronger and more effective with every passing day' 'My body is learning how to use my medical treatment more effectively; I need less and less 'X' to produce the same effect' (**Note:** It is dangerous to change or reduce medication without consulting your doctor.)

~ SUMMARY ~

Self-programming is software for your brain. It impacts on the physical, emotional and spiritual. Feel free to design it carefully.

UNIT 8

DEEP DARK SECRETS

'Am I he who would give to the world
the love I cannot give to myself?'
ANON

These words I (SC) found scribbled in the diary of a heart attack victim dated three weeks before his death.

Human beings often have aspects of themselves that they feel compelled to keep private or secret. Time and again we read in the media about public figures, church leaders, and professionals, who emerge as people with all-too-human failings! The secrets that come out include dishonesty, cheating, betrayal of trust, inadequacy, business frauds, academic failures, illicit relationships, alcoholism, drug abuse, etc. The list is endless.

Dr Dean Ornish commented: 'All of us struggle with issues that are in many ways very different, yet when we look a little deeper, we find that others' issues are not unlike our own. We have so much in common. Whatever the issue is, the fear is that we'll be rejected. So we often hide it and pretend to be something we're not – If I reveal me, what happens?'

However, current research is now demonstrating that the suppressing of deep dark secrets can precipitate or accelerate the progression of various illnesses, especially cancer. People who lead lives of secret isolation have been demonstrated to have lower immune function. Conversely, there is also research is reporting how talking about or even writing about these 'secrets' can enhance immune function and help move us towards wellness. (*See* Journalling, page 47). If you are looking to improve your health, then it would be well worthwhile choosing any unpleasant event from the past or from your current behaviour and looking to heal it. You can do this on your own or with the help of a competent counsellor or psychotherapist.

It is also useful to bear in mind that, as we go through childhood and young adulthood, events, reactions and responses are stored away in the unconscious through the eyes of, and from the perspective of a younger self. The emotions attached to these events will likely be the immature feelings we had at that time.

Even though we may have long since thought an event was resolved, those powerful emotions may still be trapped in our unconscious, potentially blocking or limiting our recovery potential. Writing or talking about these 'secrets' frees any blockage.

UNRESOLVED PAST LOSSES OR ISSUES

All of us have hopes and dreams we gather as we proceed along the road of life. Many of these will be achieved but invariably there are some which will not. These can include relationships, marriage, career, having children, travel, etc. There comes a point when the realisation dawns on us that we are not going to realise them. If the emotions of loss and grieving for these unfulfilled hopes and dreams are not expressed, these too can become a potential co-factor in the occurrence of cancer. Likewise, identifying such losses of the soul, and expressing the emotions attached to them, can form an important element in achieving healing. The occurrence of cancer itself can become the catalyst for the extinguishing of hopes and dreams and the emotions around this will demand expression.

~ SUMMARY ~

Deep dark secrets can kill. Expression of the emotions around them is healing. Effective methods are available to you to do so now.

KEY NOTES

UNIT 9

RELEASING NEGATIVE EMOTION

Resentment is like taking poison yourself, and waiting for the other person to die. If you focus on why you are angry, you will probably become angrier. If you focus on whether you wish to be angry or whether the anger is useful for learning, the anger will probably diminish.

Conventional wisdom in psychology says that negative emotions cause a narrowing in a person's thinking and acting repertoire for survival. Conversely, positive emotions bring about a widening of a person's thinking and acting repertoire. Negative emotions trigger a suppression of immune function while positive ones trigger an enhancement. Dr L.R. Derogatis, in *Journal of the American Medical Association*, said, 'Cancer patients who express anger or express upsets survive longer.' Which would you like?

Frequently, a person's personality can become dominated by a particular negative emotion (such as anger, sadness, fear, hurt or guilt). It's as though that particular emotion becomes the dominant feature in their lives. All of us know people who, much of the time, display such distinctive negative personality traits. From a psychological standpoint, what tends to cause this is a long history of recurrence. If not dealt with adequately at the time, events involving a particular emotion become 'jammed' at the unconscious level. For such a person, even a trivial event can precipitate a cascade of all the negative emotion attaching to similar events from the past. Ordinary everyday emotions, such as anger, can suddenly become rage, sadness can become depression, and fear can become extreme anxiety.

Extremes of specific negative emotions have become identified with particular diseases, e.g. anger has become associated with heart disease, and guilt and depression with cancer. In seeking to tip the balance in the direction of health, the healing of such past events and repressed emotions is essential. However, the typical cancer patient does not have the time to engage in lengthy counselling or therapy. This is where forms of 'brief' therapy come in – psychological processes which can enable patients to release unresolved negative emotion at the unconscious level in a matter of hours without having to explore each and every related event in the past. Time Line Therapy, a form of Cognitive Behavioural

Therapy (*See* page 201) developed by Dr. Tad James, is an example of such a process. Though Field Therapy has proved particularly effective when dealing with anxiety and trauma (*See* page 199). Such interventions are best done with a qualified psychotherapist or counsellor. However, if you are negatively affected by such powerful negative emotions, it is well worth the effort to clear them out as they are blocks to recovery.

~ SUMMARY ~

Unresolved or trapped negative emotion from the past can be released and free up self-healing.

KEY NOTES

'Because I had learned how to do self-hypnosis and how to deal with pain, this cancer operation seemed so much easier than the one before. Talking to people who had the same illness helped greatly . . . ' *N.C., Dublin*

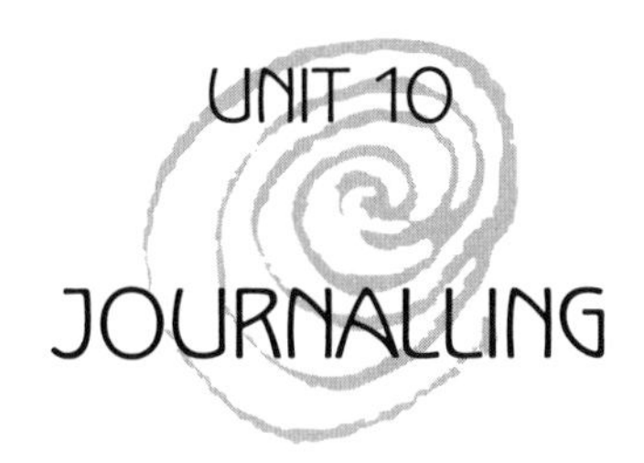

UNIT 10
JOURNALLING

Dr. James Pennebaker has spent many years studying the relationship between physical and psychological well-being and the ability to share feelings. His research revealed that repressing negative emotions, such as anger, fear, hurt or guilt, promotes unhealthy conditions in the body, and that the expression of feelings, especially through writing, has a measurable and significant effect on immune function. This effect lasts long after the writing has ceased, as shown by increased numbers of T cells (white cells in the body which are known to fight cancer and infections) and better general health.

This therapeutic process is the ideal antidote to the 'Type C coping style' that Lydia Temoshok describes in her research. She discovered that those who were emotional 'imploders', those who did not express or let out emotions were more susceptible to cancer, and those cancers progressed more rapidly than in patients who expressed emotion.

Do you have emotional 'baggage' it would be useful to off-load? Are there unresolved events in your past or in your present life which trigger strong negative emotions in you?

By writing a journal about some particular traumatic event or series of events, in the structured way described here, giving details not just the facts of what occurred, but also your feelings about it, a change takes place. As new insights are gained, an event that once triggered strong negative emotions is seen in a different light, and a feeling of calm acceptance develops.

THE PENNEBAKER PROCESS

1. Find somewhere quiet and peaceful where you won't be disturbed.
2. Begin writing about a negative event (or series of events) that seems most significant to you. This may relate to any event or time in your past, from birth to now. Write about your 'secret' or any theme relating to this.
3. Keep the pen going for at least twenty minutes – the pen should not stop or come off the page. Even if you run out of things to write about, write about that!

4. Stop after twenty minutes. You may have much more to write, but there is always tomorrow.
5. Repeat the process the following day, for a total of five days.
6. If other events come up, note them down – then leave them. You can come back and repeat this process, but stay with one event or theme at a time.
7. Make sure you write both the facts and the emotions or feelings you experienced:
   - at the time (as though you are back there right now)
   - from today's perspective (looking back on that younger you)
   - from the perspective of a detached observer – e.g. news reporter

Feel free to just scribble. Keep writing. Ignore rules about grammar, spelling, composition or sentence structure. The only person to see this is you. Discuss in written words your deepest thoughts and feelings. Write about any event... ideally the one you may have kept private or secret. Allow the story to unfold rather than construct it; the sequence and order is not important. It is critical to let go and allow your deepest emotions and thoughts.

You may find the process irritating or annoying at first, as it is so different to a 'normal' structured approach. However, there is no 'RIGHT' way to do this process.

Process Author: Dr. James Pennebaker, Ph.D. (Southern Methodist University, Dallas)

Dr Pennebaker observes, 'This form of writing does not necessarily help a person to feel better right away. In fact, the individual may feel more anxiety or depression for a while. However as insights are reached, the bad feelings lift dramatically. Things may get worse before they get better – but they always get better if you persist'.

As you proceed through the week, other traumatic or emotional events may come up. Just keep a note of them for another time and then continue. Your objective is to heal one event or period in your life.

Keep your notes in a private place – they are not for sharing with family members. As it is not useful to read over your notes after writing, you might like to burn them after each session, lest you forget where they are hidden. If you have insights in the course of writing, however, you might consider reviewing them with a professional counsellor or therapist as this has been shown to further enhance immune function.

~ SUMMARY ~

You can enhance the effectiveness of your immune system through journalling.

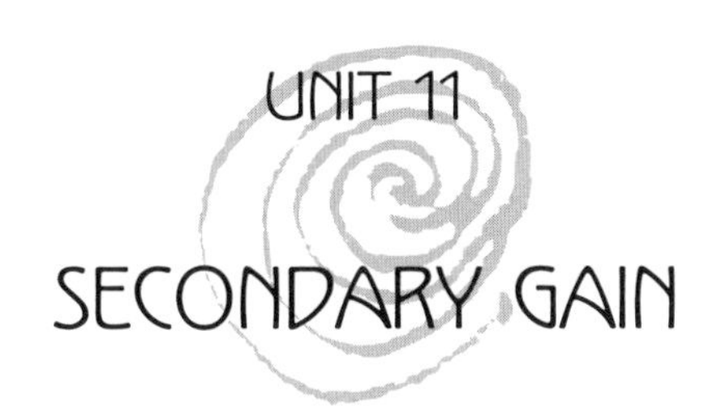

UNIT 11

SECONDARY GAIN

Secondary Gain can be loosely described as a reason for holding onto your problem. Now, before you rise up in indignation at the suggestion that someone would actually want to be ill, let us explore the concept further.

The unconscious mind sometimes causes us to think or act in ways that, at a logical level, seem inappropriate or even ridiculous, yet we do it anyway. However, it is suggested that all behaviours are thinking patterns that were once useful in some context. For instance, someone wrestling for years with the problem of excess weight might, at an unconscious level, have several valid reasons for holding on to it. Without the weight, that person might be expected to engage in intimate relationships, play sports or go dancing. At a conscious level, the person wants these things, but there may be deep-seated reasons why the unconscious will block that individual from losing weight until the root cause or some unfulfilled need has been addressed. A person with agoraphobia might appear to lead a very restricted life. However, when they have let go of the fear, they also let go of a comfortable support system: the spouse won't have to come home early to keep them company and the children won't have to do the shopping!

Illness frequently brings unexpected and unconscious rewards. Think back to a time (perhaps in childhood) when some vaguely unpleasant event was looming – say, exams – and suddenly you developed the 'flu' or an earache. The symptoms were unpleasant, but the gain, both in parental attention and in avoiding the dreaded event, was worth the pain!

These symptoms are not fabricated; they are very real – a solution that is invented outside of your conscious awareness. The unconscious finds a way of having some need met for you. So, the question to ask might be, 'If the problem or illness were to disappear, what would I lose?'

In past Behavioural Medicine programmes, we have had the participants discuss ways in which their condition has, inadvertently, begun to fill previously unmet needs in their life. Generally with a group of ten to fifteen people, we can fill 2 to 3 pages of flip-chart paper! 'I no longer have to do all the housework.', 'I get some attention at home now.', 'My boss has stopped pushing me around.', 'My mother listens to me now.' . . . And so on.

If your unconscious mind sees that the condition enables you to have certain important needs met, it will see no logic in helping to have the condition disappear! Frequently, just the process of exploring the concept of Secondary Gain causes it as a problem to disappear because you are now free to identify other ways of meeting these needs.

Dr. Carl Simonton comments, 'Many people punish themselves and others through illness and sometimes even death. Because of social and cultural conditioning, people often find it impossible to resolve stressful problems in a healthy way and therefore choose – consciously or unconsciously – to get sick as a way out.'

THINGS TO CONSIDER

- What might the condition now allow you to do (that you've always wanted to do)?
- What might the condition now stop you from having to do (that you've despised doing)?
- What does the condition allow others (family members) to do (that they've always really wanted to do)?
- What does the condition stop others from having to do (that they've privately despised doing)?

~ SUMMARY ~

Diseases and side effects can inadvertently become useful.
This is a dangerous game and can be reversed.

KEY NOTES

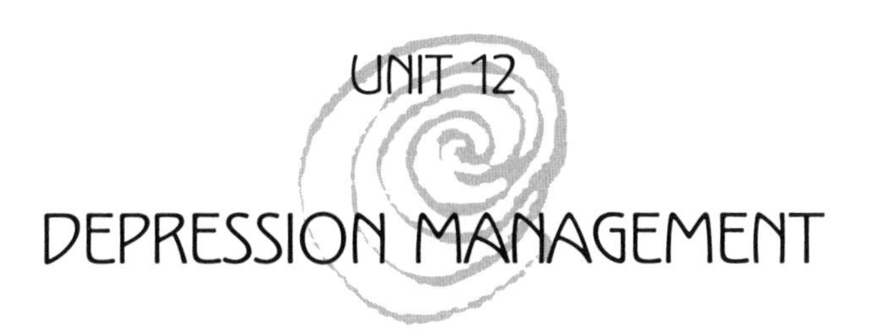

UNIT 12

DEPRESSION MANAGEMENT

'My private image of myself is very different from the image which I try to create in the minds of others in order that they may love me.'
W.H. AUDEN

Depression for many patients is part and parcel of dealing with a life-threatening or 'quality-of-life'-threatening illness. They may try to deny that they are depressed, or will perceive it as a sign of weakness to be hidden from the world. Depression has sometimes been described as a hiding place when things become too much to bear. Animals, when they are sick, retreat into quiet and dark places. Humans are not all that different.

Dr David Servan-Schreiber, clinical professor at the University of Pittsburgh School of Medicine, suggests that cancer may manifest first as a depression rather than as physical symptoms.

However, if you are determined to fight back and encourage self-healing in your body, you can't afford the luxury of leaving depression unrecognised or unaddressed. Depression, if left untreated, tends to become worse and will begin to absorb much of your thinking-time and energy.

There is no presupposition here that you ought to become depressed if you are dealing with a disease. Many people experience illness as a challenge and they rise to meet it. However, depression is sufficiently common and, potentially, such a drain on your physical and emotional resources as to demand serious consideration in any fight-back programme.

SYMPTOMS OF DEPRESSION – A CHECK-LIST

- I regularly experience depressed moods and feelings.
- I get no pleasure from things I normally enjoy.
- I have difficulty concentrating.
- I have no interest in my normal hobbies or pastimes.

- I wake too early and can't get back to sleep.
- I find it hard to make decisions.
- I'm not performing efficiently at work.
- I have no inclination for sex or intimacy.
- My appetite is poor.
- I can't look forward to the future with any sense of pleasure.
- I get frequent headaches.
- I can't even enjoy watching television or doing a crossword.
- I find mornings are the worst.
- I'm tearful at times and have no control over this.
- I feel I can't cope.
- I feel guilty for having nothing I can justifiably complain about.
- The feeling that I ought to be able to 'get a grip' makes me feel worse.
- The thoughts of a holiday leave me cold.
- I've even thought of taking my life.
- I'm tired all the time – and I'm not on medication for my condition.

A diagnosis of depression should only be made by a trained health professional, doctor, clinical psychologist or psychiatrist although studies reveal that depression is missed in the doctor's office more often than it is identified. However, if you can strongly identify with more than five or six of the above, then it may be time to get some professional help to assess if you are depressed, as this depression can suppress your immune function.

Dealing with a serious illness absorbs a lot of time, and your time is precious. Seeking professional help will ensure that you have the physical and emotional energy to engage in a fight-back programme. Taking appropriate anti-depression medication is not a sign of failure or weakness. It is just plain common sense when engaged in a proactive response to illness. If you had a broken leg, would you decline a cast?

~ SUMMARY ~

Depression has been shown to be a potential causal agent in the occurrence of cancer and in its progression. You cannot afford the luxury of undiagnosed depression.

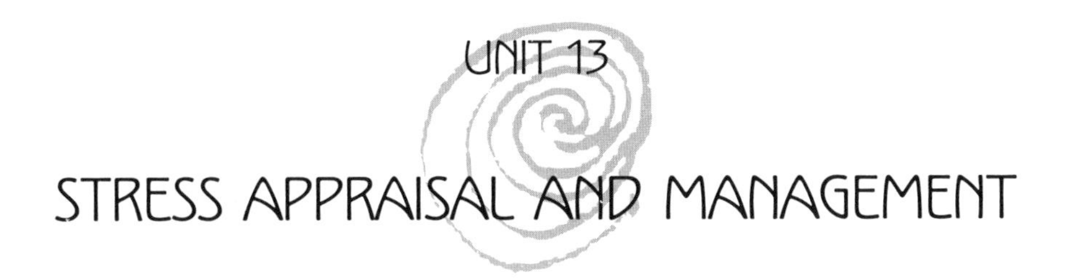

UNIT 13

STRESS APPRAISAL AND MANAGEMENT

'My crown is in my heart, not on my head;
Not decked with diamonds and Indian stones, nor to be seen;
My crown is called content;
A crown it is that seldom kings enjoy.'
WILLIAM SHAKESPEARE, *HENRY VI*, PART III

THE STRESS RESPONSE

There are two types of stress. One is acute or sudden and the body has reserves of chemicals or hormones such as adrenaline (epinephrine) to deal with this. However, if a stressor becomes chronic or long term, the system becomes exhausted. Dr Hans Selye, the father of modern stress theory, and Founder of the Canadian Institute of Stress, suggested that the stages of the stress response are alarm, resistance, coping, exhaustion and recovery.

FOR A PATIENT, THE POTENTIAL STRESSORS ARE:

- The actually diagnosis (the moment of diagnosis itself!)
- Treatment of the medical condition (surgery, chemotherapy, radiotherapy, etc.)
- The side-effects of treatment
- Personal perception of the diagnosis and ongoing situation, e.g. 'Will I die?' 'What does this mean?'
- Pre-existing physical, emotional, behavioural and spiritual stressors
- Stress has been clearly shown to compromise immune function. Prolonged unrelenting stress massively compromises it. Disease and treatment, depending on the individual's personal sense of control, cause massive protracted stress and this stress is often missed or ignored in the conventional medical model!

- In itself, stress is neither good nor bad – in fact, without challenge and stress, the body and mind tend to deteriorate. The stress response is part of our evolved survival mechanism. When the body encounters stress, or perceived stress, hormones flood into the bloodstream which causes the following to happen:
  - Heart rate goes up
  - Respiration goes up
  - Blood pressure goes up
  - Triglycerides go up
  - Platelet aggregation goes up
  - Blood flow to skeletal muscles goes up
  - Muscular tension goes up, metabolism
  - Speeds up, pupils dilate
  - Body may perspire
  - Blood is channelled away from peripheral areas – which is why you may become pale
  - Digestion begins to shut down.

Firstly, there is direct suppression of immune function by the stress hormones such as adrenalin (epinephrine) and noradrenalin (norepinephrine) released from the adrenal glands. They suppress the levels of killer T cells, the body's first line of defence. Next, these hormones cause the thymus to shrink, killing immune cells, or leading to their release at a premature (weaker) stage of development. Beta-endorphins, activated by the hypothalamus, suppress immune cell activity as well as acting as the body's natural painkillers.

This response prepares the body, in seconds, to prepare for what has become known as the 'Fight or Flight' response. The maximum response is triggered by a threat to your survival. This state will continue as long as heightened readiness or actual action is required which, of course, has a lot to do with how you perceive the situation. When the threat has passed, the body returns to normal. This normalisation is triggered by the release of cortisol, which, although it moves the body back towards normal balance (homeostasis), it also suppresses the immune system.

In the case of a patient receiving a serious diagnosis/prognosis, the threat does not pass, and depending on the individual and their personal coping style, the body may stay in a state of high alert and hormonal chaos, shown in research to lead, potentially, to: high resting heart rate, heart disease, platelet aggregation, reactive

The Stress Response
PERCEPTION OF THREAT

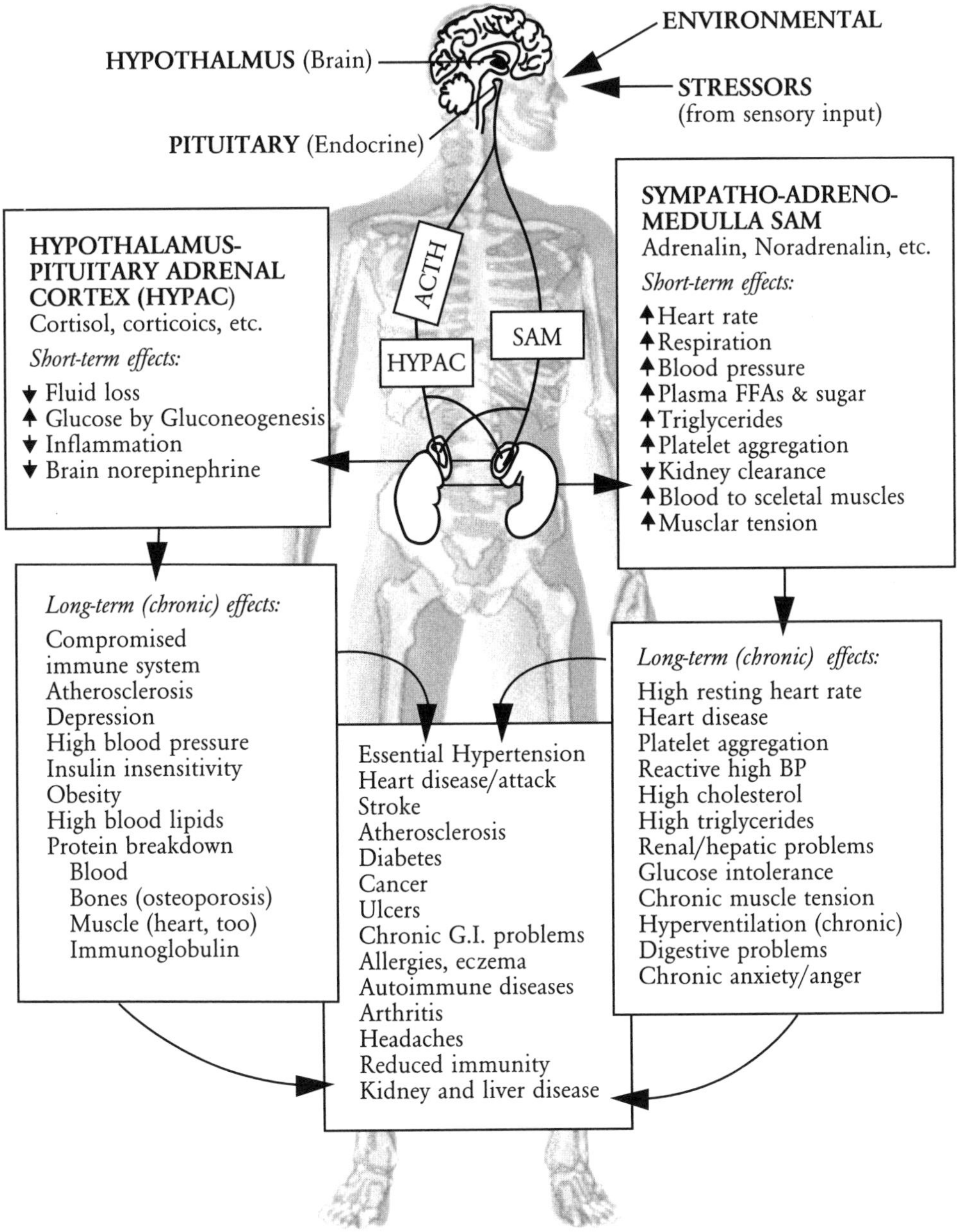

ENVIRONMENTAL

HYPOTHALMUS (Brain)

STRESSORS
(from sensory input)

PITUITARY (Endocrine)

ACTH

HYPAC

SAM

HYPOTHALAMUS-PITUITARY ADRENAL CORTEX (HYPAC)
Cortisol, corticoics, etc.

Short-term effects:

- ↓ Fluid loss
- ↑ Glucose by Gluconeogenesis
- ↓ Inflammation
- ↓ Brain norepinephrine

SYMPATHO-ADRENO-MEDULLA SAM
Adrenalin, Noradrenalin, etc.

Short-term effects:

- ↑ Heart rate
- ↑ Respiration
- ↑ Blood pressure
- ↑ Plasma FFAs & sugar
- ↑ Triglycerides
- ↑ Platelet aggregation
- ↓ Kidney clearance
- ↑ Blood to sceletal muscles
- ↑ Musclar tension

Long-term (chronic) effects:

Compromised immune system
Atherosclerosis
Depression
High blood pressure
Insulin insensitivity
Obesity
High blood lipids
Protein breakdown
  Blood
  Bones (osteoporosis)
  Muscle (heart, too)
  Immunoglobulin

Essential Hypertension
Heart disease/attack
Stroke
Atherosclerosis
Diabetes
Cancer
Ulcers
Chronic G.I. problems
Allergies, eczema
Autoimmune diseases
Arthritis
Headaches
Reduced immunity
Kidney and liver disease

Long-term (chronic) effects:

High resting heart rate
Heart disease
Platelet aggregation
Reactive high BP
High cholesterol
High triglycerides
Renal/hepatic problems
Glucose intolerance
Chronic muscle tension
Hyperventilation (chronic)
Digestive problems
Chronic anxiety/anger

high blood pressure, high cholesterol, high triglycerides, glucose intolerance, chronic muscle tension, chronic hyperventilation, digestive problems, and chronic anxiety and anger.

This 'stuck' state can lead to poor immune-system function, depression, insulin insensitivity and more, which research has shown can lead to: heart disease, heart attack, stroke, atherosclerosis, diabetes, cancer, ulcers, autoimmune diseases, arthritis, headaches, as well as kidney and liver disease.

For the newly diagnosed poorly-coping patient, this is what can appear on the horizon, and this is before treatment for the cancer has even begun! Minimal attention is currently given to the impact of such chronic stress and its proven negative effect on the mind and body. Dr Richard Earle, President of the Canadian Institute of Stress, suggests that 'The longer and more intense a stress reaction, the more wear and tear is inflicted on the body.' The emerging fields of behavioural medicine and psychoneuroimmunology are seeking to correct this situation and provide patients with additional tools for stress awareness and management.

Emotions, behaviours, and life events are constantly influencing the hormonal mixture in the bloodstream. If you are threatened, the body releases among others, the hormone called adrenaline. When the threat passes, other hormones are released to cancel out the alert. Similarly, if a doctor were to inject adrenaline into your bloodstream, your body/mind would go into a state of high alert.

Scientists suggest that up to 80% of modern man's diseases are psychosomatic or stress related. Our automatic stress-response causes the heart rate to shoot up, blood pressure then soars, the stomach and intestines stop all the busy activity of digestion, hearing and smell become more acute. Hundreds of other physical changes occur without our even knowing it. With stress comes a sharp increase in energy consumption. The reaction puts the entire body in a state of readiness, and whether the cause of the stress is inside the body or outside, it will often cause a person to become completely drained.

Short-term stress is part and parcel of modern living. However, a serious disease represents a source of long term or chronic stress. The body responses can become habituated or conditioned to being in permanent high alert and which exhausts an already challenged body (and spirit).

Does this sound like how you want to feel when you need to trigger a healing response? Probably not! Serious illness can cause enormous, and frequently ongoing, stresses to the body. Our objective here is to encourage you to consider what stress is, what causes it, and how you can best manage it to enhance your healing response.

TEN COMMON RULES OF STRESS MANAGEMENT

- Set aside a daily time for reflection, meditation and relaxation.
- Set goals and priorities, and avoid conflicting goals.
- Find support groups, and rid yourself of negative influences around you.
- Take care of your body.
- Learn to manage and organise yourself and your time.
- Set aside the things that you can't control.
- Dwell on your positive aspects and talents.
- Learn how to say 'NO'.
- Indulge in stress-free entertainment and hobbies.
- Find solace and peace in your spiritual life.

WHAT ACTUALLY STRESSES YOU?

Ongoing stressful events/people/situations?

1. ______________________________
2. ______________________________
3. ______________________________

How do you cope? What do you do?

1. ______________________________
2. ______________________________
3. ______________________________

Stressful events/people/situations during the past few months?

1. ______________________________
2. ______________________________
3. ______________________________

How did you cope? What did you do?

1. ______________________________
2. ______________________________
3. ______________________________

FIVE WAYS TO EXAMINE STRESSFUL SITUATIONS

1. Do you have some control over the stressor?
2. Is the stressor controlled by someone or something else?
3. Is it important to your life or professional goals?
4. Is it better to leave this alone?
5. Are benefits of dealing with the stressor greater than the stress it will create?

TWELVE WAYS TO REDUCE STRESS

1. Physical activity

When you are nervous, angry or upset, release the pressure through exercise or physical activity. Running, walking, playing tennis, swimming or working in the garden are just some of the activities you can do. Physical exercise will relieve that uptight feeling and relax you. Remember, the body and mind work together! Even if you are capable of only tiny movements due to your condition, that is enough – as long as you do it daily!

2. Share your stress

It helps to talk to someone about your concerns and worries. A friend, family member, teacher, or counsellor can help you to see your problem in a different light. If you feel your problem is serious, seek professional help. Knowing when to ask will help you avoid serious problems later on.

3. Know your limits

If a problem is beyond your control and can't be changed right now, don't fight the situation. Learn to accept it for the moment, until such time as you can take steps to change it.

4. Take care of yourself

you are special. Get enough rest and eat well. If you are irritable from lack of sleep, or if you are not eating correctly, you will have less ability to deal with stressful situations. If stress repeatedly keeps you from sleeping, you should seek help.

5. Make time for fun

Schedule time for both work and recreation. Play can be just as important to your well being as work. Take a break from your daily routine to just relax and have fun.

6. Be a participant

One way to keep from becoming bored, sad and lonely, is to go where it is all happening; sitting alone by yourself can leave you more frustrated, sad and lonely. Instead of feeling sorry for yourself, get involved and become a participant. Offer your services in some neighbourhood activity or volunteer organisations. Help yourself by helping other people. Get involved in the world and the people around you, and you will find they will be attracted to you.

7. Check off your tasks

Trying to take care of everything at once can seem overwhelming and, as a result, you may not accomplish anything. Instead, make a list of the tasks you have to do, then do them one at a time, checking them off as they're completed. Give priority to the most important ones and do those first. You don't have to finish the list.

8. Must you always be right?

Do other people upset you, particularly when they don't do things your way? Try co-operation instead of confrontation; it's better then fighting. A little give and take on both sides will reduce the strain and can surprise you by making you both feel better.

9. It's OK to cry

A good cry can be a healthy way to bring relief to your anxiety, and it might even prevent a headache or other physical consequences. Take some deep breaths; they also release tension. Russian researchers showed that tears enhance immune function.

10. Create an inner quiet scene

You can't always run away, but you can 'dream the impossible dream'. A quiet country scene painted in your mind's eye or on canvas, can temporarily take you out of the turmoil of a stressful situation. Change the focus by reading a good book or playing beautiful music to create a sense of peace and tranquillity.

11. Avoid self-medication

Although you can use prescribed drugs or modest amounts of alcohol to relieve stress temporarily – and they can be useful in taking you through a rough patch – they do not change the conditions that caused the stress in the first place. It will still be waiting.

12. Learn the art of relaxation

The best strategy is the method that works best for you. A relaxation response can be conditioned, according to Professor Herbert Benson, in a matter of weeks.

~ SUMMARY ~

Your level of stress-hardiness or resilience
can be re-conditioned by you.

THE LIFE STRESS TEST

Holmes and Rahe Social Readjustment Scale

The scale lists forty-three common life changes in the order in which they have been found to be predictions of illness. The research of Holmes and Rahe showed that if a person experiences an excessive amount of stressors within a set time period in their life, they have a greatly raised probability of developing a serious condition, hence the importance for the patient going through the experience of a life-threatening disease and its treatment.

However, in this section, we are looking at overloading of stressors. To find your score, simply write in the values of the items in the following list that apply to you within the past year. Then add up your score and compare it with the range of scores that are given at the end of the test.

Do bear in mind, however, that it is not the stressor itself that is significant here, but rather our perception of it. So, many people with extra-high scores might well escape unscathed.

Rank	Event	Value	Your Score
1	Death of spouse	100	________
2	Divorce	73	________
3	Marital problems	65	________
4	Jail term	63	________
5	Death of a close family member	63	________
6	Personal injury or illness	53	________
7	Marriage	50	________
8	Fired from work	47	________
9	Marital reconciliation	45	________
10	Retirement	45	________
11	Change in family member's health	44	________
12	Pregnancy	40	________
13	Sexual difficulties	39	________
14	Addition to family	39	________
15	Business readjustments	39	________
16	Change in financial status	38	________
17	Death of close friend	37	________
18	Change to different line of work	36	________

19	Change in number of marital arguments	35	________
20	Mortgage or loan over €100,000	31	________
21	Foreclosure of mortgage/loan house cost approx €80,000)	30	________
22	Change in work responsibilities	29	________
23	Son or daughter leaving home	29	________
24	Trouble with in-laws	29	________
25	Outstanding personal achievement	28	________
26	Spouse begins or stops work	26	________
27	Starting or finishing school	26	________
28	Change in living conditions	25	________
29	Revision of personal habits	24	________
30	Trouble with boss	23	________
31	Change in work hours/conditions	20	________
32	Change in residence	20	________
33	Change in schools	20	________
34	Change in recreational habits	19	________
35	Change in Church activities	19	________
36	Change in social activities	19	________
37	Mortgage or loan under €100,000	17	________
38	Change in sleeping habits	16	________
39	Change in number of family gatherings	15	________
40	Change in eating habits	15	________
41	Vacation	13	________
42	Christmas season	12	________
43	Minor violation of the law	11	________
	TOTAL		________

Total score less than 150: 37% chance of illness during next 2 years
150 to 300: 51% chance of illness
Over 300: 80% chance of serious illness

~ SUMMARY ~

Stress responses accumulate in the body and the mind and reach a critical mass point where they can lead to diseases such as cancer.

UNIT 14

PRIORITIES AND RESOURCE MANAGEMENT

For most of us, our principal resources include: personal attributes, skills, time, energy, money confidence, family, friends, colleagues and personal relationships. All of these, inevitably, come under strain when you are dealing with a significant illness. Patients sometimes, inadvertently, squander or misuse the most precious of these resources, perhaps trying at some unconscious level to 'prove' that they are not sick.

TIME

If you have been diagnosed with an illness, then the clock is ticking. Many people, at the actual time they are diagnosed, feel physically healthy – apart from some unexpected pain, a lump, or perhaps blood where there shouldn't be blood. In other words, they may be 98% well, and only 2% ill. Up to the moment of diagnosis, the person's body was in reasonable shape. However, we know that diagnosis often triggers a drop in immune function. We also know that diagnosis can cause patients to slip into an 'illness' mind-set making matters worse. In no time at all, they are acting like ill people. Illness has become their 'identity'.

The best time to think about responding in a structured and proactive fashion is immediately you get your diagnosis or confirmation, although we believe it is virtually never too late. This is a time when, physically and psychologically, you are probably still in good shape. You can start crafting an optimum environment in which your body's 'fight-back' mechanism (the immune system) can function effectively. Late-stage intervention with Behavioural Medicine has proved to be useful in prolonging life by an average of two years, according to some studies in Europe and the USA (Spiegel, 1989 and Eysenck and Grossarth-Maticek, 1990, 1991). However, its effectiveness in improving quality of life makes it well worthwhile. How much more powerful is early intervention, can only be surmised.

ENERGY

When people have cancer, they will often receive powerful and toxic medical treatments. Physical and emotional energy will tend to be in short supply. As therapists, we are appalled at how many clients, in an effort to maintain the 'status quo', will resist taking time out for rest or for naps. We see patients exhausting themselves looking after children or ageing parents, doing shopping, often trying to act 'well' so as to shield a partner or spouse from worry or hassle. This is ridiculous! Like in Las Vegas, if you over-spend, you don't get to stay in the game – you have to earn or gather to get to stay! We love the quote from John O'Donohue, 'A day is over and so much of it was wasted on things that meant so little to you, duties and meetings from which your heart was absent. You mistake the insistent pressure of daily demands for reality, and your more delicate and intuitive nature wilts.'

Under normal circumstances, the body rebuilds itself when we sleep. When ill, we need even more sleep and rest. This is the time to be absolutely uncompromising in prioritising; this is the time to 'nap' outrageously! I am amazed at how often patients will refuse to put-off visitors or social engagements even though they are emotionally or physically 'running on empty'. When autumn winds come, the branches carrying the most foliage are the most at risk. The wind will always come; you just don't know when or how strong it will be.

CONFIDENCE

Years ago I purchased a book just for the title: *You Can't Afford the Luxury of a Negative Thought, a book for people with any life threatening illness – including life*, by John Roger and Peter McWilliams. When health-threatened, we need all the confidence we can get; Confidence in ourselves, our bodies, our doctors, our medical treatment, our prognosis, and our recovery capabilities. Negativity has a high price if not balanced by confidence.

RELATIONSHIPS

Social support and interaction have been shown in numerous studies to improve immune function and recovery prospects. However, the onset of illness puts great pressures on relationships and in so doing threatens these relationships at the very time when they are most important for recovery. Patients frequently retreat from social activities, not wanting to be a 'wet blanket'. Loved ones often have a hard time dealing with the effects of the emotional maelstrom that many patients find themselves in.

In implementing an effective recovery programme, it is vital to move towards positive, supportive people and activities, rather than away from them. Often, even friends and family will tend to move away from ill people because they do not understand the illness. Perhaps they are frightened themselves or feel helpless, not knowing how to be of support.

In a 'fight-back' situation, it is essential for you the patient to let people know how they can help with shopping, cleaning, finance, talking, etc. It is amazing how positive friends and relatives become when you make it clear how, specifically, they can support you; it helps them deal with their own sense of helplessness.

Numerous studies have shown that participation in support groups improves immune function so, even if you don't like the idea, be 'selfish' and look for a support group now.

CARING FOR YOUR SUPPORT CREW

Psychologist William James said 'We crave to be appreciated.' Every time NASA launch the space shuttle, perhaps just four or five astronauts go up, but they will have a support crew of hundreds. In tackling a significant illness, you too need such a support crew. However, they need care and maintenance also.

We would ask you some questions:

- Do you have a support crew?
- Do you let them get close to you?
- When did you last say to one of them 'I need your care/loving/support/help?
- When did you last thank them?
- When did you last tell them how important they are?
- What is it that you really appreciate about them? (specifically)
- Do you actually know simple things about them?
- How do they like to spend their time?
- What are their hopes and dreams?
- What are their biggest and deepest concerns or worries in life?
- What is their favourite food, flower or colour?
- When did you last do something for them, a surprise, without precedent, to let them know they are appreciated?
- How can you show or tell them that you value them, in a way that is meaningful to them?
- Do you feel free to tell them when you do 'not' want their help?

Right now might be a useful time to let your support crew know that they are important too, and that you understand what they are going through also, and that you really cherish them. The beneficiary will be you.

MONEY

We are regularly amazed at patients who will carry heavy bags of shopping and queue for a bus, or sit in a traffic-jam driving to their GP, just to avoid spending 5–10 euro on a taxi fare even though, financially, they can well afford it. When you are life-threatened, you need to decide which is more important, energy or money. Money can be replaced – you can't! It is essential that you at least consider and review how you allocate expenditure of money, as opposed to time, as part of your recovery programme. You are looking to create an optimum environment for your body.

Chronic worries about money suppress immunity – so go and talk to someone. We frequently sit with patients who are agonising over mounting medical bills and worrying if their health insurance will cover them. We ask the question, 'Who will be spending your money if you die?' So, why not invest it in living now!

~ SUMMARY ~

When dealing with a major illness, you have exceptional demands on you. This is a time to have a precise strategy for managing your resources carefully.

KEY NOTES

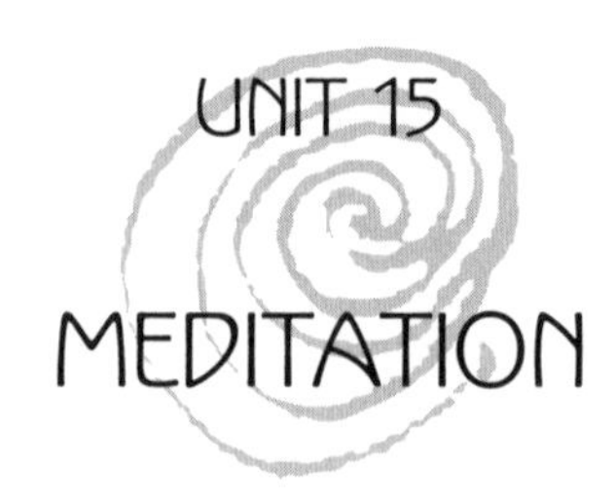

UNIT 15

MEDITATION

Meditation is the process of gently quietening the mind. When your mind is quiet, you feel peaceful. Any sense of separateness and isolation from the world tends to disappear. Current research indicates that the regular practice of any one of a wide variety of meditation techniques can significantly improve the performance of your immune system, reduce stress and tension, and improve the prospects of remission or cure. Researchers at the University of Miami found that daily meditation increased both the activity and numbers of immune cells. In a three-year study, involving elderly residents of a nursing home, those who meditated were all alive at the end of the study as opposed to only 38% of the non-meditators.

Professor Herbert Benson at Harvard University has been carrying out clinical trials of meditation since the early 1970s, also showing measurable improvements. Jon Kabat-Zinn, PhD., has been running a hospital-based eight-week meditation programme at the University of Massachusetts Medical Centre for more than twenty years. Studies of his work show that those meditating report significantly reduced pain levels and fewer side-effects from their treatment. In 1990, Dr Dean Ornish, a Harvard graduate cardiologist, was the first person to show conclusively that heart disease could be reversed; his reversal programme includes meditation as a major component.

MEDITATION IS NOW WIDELY USED TO:

- Improve immune function (the 'fight back' system in the body).
- Reduce the symptoms of illness such as sleep problems, anxiety, etc.
- Manage the side effects of treatment (tablets, chemotherapy, radiotherapy, surgery, etc.)
- Improve emotional well-being.
- Increase the likelihood of remission or cure.

Meditation can be used anywhere (train, bus etc.) even on the way to work, and can be learned in one easy session. It is usable by anyone, regardless of age, religion or beliefs.

THE BENSON MEDITATION TECHNIQUE

The 'Relaxation Response' is a simple yet powerful form of private meditation developed, during the early 1970s, by Dr Herbert Benson, M.D., a Professor of Medicine at Harvard Medical School. He is also Director of the Division of Behavioural Medicine and the Hypertension Unit at Boston's Beth Israel Hospital.

Instructions

1. Select a quiet calm environment with as few distractions as possible. Sit quietly and close your eyes, focusing on your breathing for a few moments to 'arrive' at what you are about to do, leaving aside the intrusions of everyday life for these next 20 minutes.
2. An upright sitting posture (not lying down) is important, so that there is no undue muscular tension in your body. You should be comfortable and relaxed. Avoid crossing your legs or intertwining your fingers as this can interfere with blood circulation or result in cramping. Remember, when the body relaxes, its temperature will tend to fall slightly, so make sure you are in a warm environment with adequate clothing.
3. With your eyes closed, start repeating the word 'ONE' (or any other word or phrase of your choice) to yourself, silently or aloud. This repetition encourages the mind to stop wandering and helps stem the constant train of different thoughts that normally pass through the mind. Allow your body to breathe easily and naturally. Continue repeating the word for 15-20 minutes. You may open your eyes to check the time, but do not use an alarm.
4. Refrain from worrying about how well you are performing the technique. When distracting thoughts intrude (as they will), just gently let them go . . . and return to the repetition of the word. This passive attitude is the most important element in producing the Relaxation Response. When thoughts present themselves, and you become aware of them, just acknowledge them as 'Just thinking!' and return your focus to the repetition of your chosen word.
5. The objective is not to force a deep level of relaxation. It is to allow relaxation to occur. Simply maintain a passive attitude and let it happen. With practice, the Relaxation Response will come with little effort.
6. When you finish, sit quietly for a few moments, at first with your eyes closed and then with your eyes open. When you stand up, do so gently.

Practice the Benson Meditation Technique at least once (ideally twice) each day but not within two hours after any meal, since it has been shown that digestion interferes with Relaxation Response. Avoid practising just before going to bed.

This is only one of a wide variety of meditation techniques that you could use. Meditation forms an important part of Buddhist teaching, and it is perfectly possible to learn their particular techniques without becoming a Buddhist monk. Equally, in the last thirty years there has been a resurgence within the Christian Church (the Catholic Church in particular), of meditation and contemplative prayer, largely as the result of the writings and teaching of Fr. John Main.

Remember, you can derive benefit from meditation without necessarily believing in it or liking it. There is no such thing as bad meditation. Any meditation is beneficial in calming the mind and bringing us in deeper connection with the workings of the mind and body.

Benefits of the Benson Meditation Technique:

- Improves immune function.
- Relieves fatigue and helps you cope with subconscious anxieties
- Reduces the stress that can lead to high blood pressure, hardening of the arteries, heart attack or stroke.
- Improves your ability to relax, both physically and mentally.
- Reduces the frequency and/or intensity of headaches and also angina and arthritis pain.
- Useful in the treatment of lower back pain.
- Helps regulate cardiac arrhythmias.
- Reduces the severity of nausea/vomiting with chemotherapy.
- Reduces the tendency towards compulsive smoking, eating and alcohol abuse.
- Can help greatly with insomnia and sleep problems.
- Helps conserve the body's store of energy.
- Makes you more alert so you can focus on what's important.
- Often reduces cholesterol levels without the need for drugs.
- Can increase HDL (good cholesterol).
- Can reduce reliance on prescription drugs.
- Has no unpleasant side effects.
- No educational requirement or aptitude is necessary.

~ SUMMARY ~

Medical Meditation is an evidence-based method of stress-management.

KEY NOTES

'I benefited greatly from the emotional support I received from the sympathetic style of leadership and teaching by Sean Collins at a time in my recovery from cancer when I felt most vulnerable. Practical ways of handling stress, many of which were new to me, were also beneficial. I was also encouraged by the personal contributions from individuals in the group which I could relate to, and I appreciated the confidentiality that was always emphasised.'
J. McC., Co. Dublin

UNIT 16

VISUALISATION AND POSITIVE IMAGING

Visualisation is the process by which we form images or pictures in the mind's eye. As children, we do this automatically. Many youngsters of five, six or seven will readily imagine their favourite TV programme, complete with imaginary screen, if it is suggested to them in the right way. As adults, we still visualise as we process information but, as most people do this unconsciously, we need a little time and practice to bring the mental pictures into conscious awareness.

Images are very useful and adaptable things, and can become a representation or metaphor for those parts of our bodies that are affected by an illness and for the illness itself. As importantly, they provide a 'target' for the unconscious mind the means by which the body can help to heal itself. The following process will develop your own healing scenario, which may be accompanied by feelings and sounds too. Remember, as you do this, that the unconscious mind and your immune system are constantly eavesdropping on your internal self-talk, be it positive or negative.

A good example of this would be a person with arthritis visualising a special lubricant flowing into the joints to loosen them. A woman with breast cancer may see her tumour as, say, a field of grass, and her immune system as the sheep grazing on it, continually 'nibbling it away'. Others may like the metaphor of a battle, seeing their cancer as an enemy army and their immune system as soldiers in their own fighting force. The most important thing is to find a set of images that suits you and feels right for you.

HOW TO VISUALISE

1. Sit down and make yourself comfortable.

2. Notice what your experience of your condition is right now, at this moment – how you feel, what you see and what you hear internally in relation to it. Allow an image to come into your mind that represents the problem.

This may be a simple image, say, of a blocked artery in the heart, or it may be a colour, a shape, an object, or a person that represents a cancer, a pain, or any other symptom. Go with whatever comes up first – however bizarre it may seem.

3. Now decide what you want to have happen to this condition: arteries to open, pain to reduce, unwanted behaviour to change, tumour to shrink, etc., and note it down briefly.
4. Now decide what has to happen for the first image to become the second: a change in colour, shape or size; soldiers killing the enemy tumour cells. You might prefer a less aggressive approach, such as a 'pied piper' charming the cancer cells away to their destruction – use whatever is right for you. Do you need to add anything to the scene to help it change, or have you got enough resources present in the picture? If there is anything else you need, add it now. Now allow the change to occur until it is completely as you would wish.
5. Now close your eyes and go through a One-Minute Body Relaxation session.

THE ONE-MINUTE BODY RELAXATION

With your eyes closed, take a deep breath, hold it briefly and exhale slowly. Then, take another deep breath, hold, and exhale slowly. Each time you breathe in, imagine you are inhaling a feeling of relaxation or some other similar 'good feeling' through your nostrils. Each time you exhale, allow that good feeling to flow to different parts of the body as follows:

- The scalp and ears
- The head and face
- The neck and both shoulders
- The left arm and hand
- The right arm and hand
- The chest and abdomen
- The back muscles, upper, middle and lower
- The left hip and left upper leg
- The left lower leg and left foot
- The right hip and upper leg
- The right lower leg and right foot
- The entire body from the top of the head down to the tips of your toes

Note: Each time you do a one-minute relaxation, you are conditioning your body and building a skill. Within a few weeks of regular practice, the body learns to do it in a matter of seconds, so don't be surprised when you find it taking less and less time to relax!

You can use visualisation as part of your self-hypnosis routine but is not essential. Many patients working with visualisation use affirmations along with their internal imaging e.g. 'The tumour is shrinking by 10 percent every day', 'My coronary arteries are opening up by 15% each week', etc.

Research suggests you do at least two sessions of visualisation a day.

Note: It is **not** essential to have crystal-clear images in your mind. The research in this area has found no differences in effect with those who are, supposedly, 'poor' image makers. Human beings are unique in the way they represent things in their minds so however you do it is perfect! Just do it.

~ SUMMARY ~

What you focus on expands. What you visualise tends to come about because the unconscious cannot tell the difference between a 'real' experience and one imagined vividly and in detail.

KEY NOTES

'The contact between members of the group gave me support and encouragement. All of this was made possible by the facilitators.' *B. O'S., Dublin*

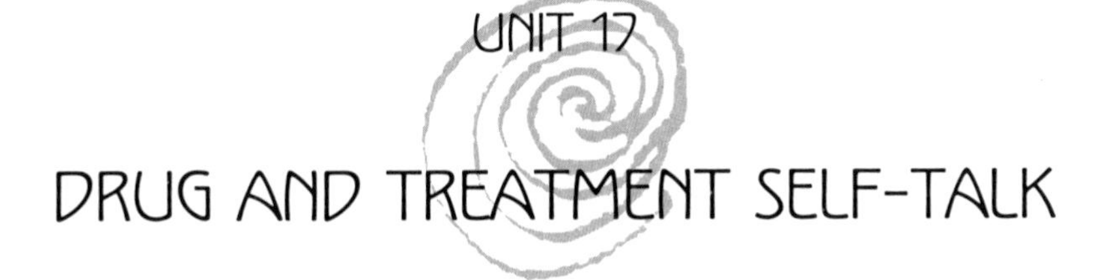

UNIT 17

DRUG AND TREATMENT SELF-TALK

Professor Paul Dorian, Professor of Medicine at the University of Toronto, was curious as to whether a person's attitude towards their medication had any significant impact on the effectiveness of their medication and on survival rates. His research was carried out with heart patients. Those who took their medications either inconsistently, or with an attitude of resentment: 'Why do I have to take this stuff?' were twice as likely to die prematurely as those who took medication regularly and with an attitude of gratitude: 'I'm lucky there is medication I can take for my problem'.

In light of the this information, it is worth reviewing your own attitude towards the medications you take and adjusting your attitude, if needs be, using self-hypnosis. What is your attitude and what are your saying to yourself when you are taking or receiving treatment?

~ SUMMARY ~

What you say to yourself when receiving treatment or taking medication can change your odds of recovery for the better or for the worse. You choose!

KEY NOTES

PART 2

PHYSICAL, BEHAVIOURAL & NUTRITIONAL

UNIT 18

BREATHING AND BREATH TRAINING

BREATHING AND WELLNESS

Without food, we die in months; without water, we die in days; without air, we die in minutes. We need air to oxygenate our blood to oxygenate the cells from which we are made.

There are 300,0000 million capillaries in the lungs. All blood passes through the lungs every minute. Every day, 10,000 litres of air pass through the lungs. You breathe 14 times a minute on average – that's 20,000 times a day. Each minute, less than one-tenth of a litre of blood flows through the top of the lungs, two-thirds of a litre flows through the middle and more than one litre flows through the bottom. The lungs are a miracle in biology!

The foundation of health is a healthy bloodstream, the vital system that transports oxygen and nutrients to every cell in your body. If you have a healthy circulatory system, you will live a long and healthy life. The key element for that system is breathing. With each breath, you can stimulate the life processes of each and every cell in your body. Breathing not only controls the oxygenation of the cells, it also partially regulates the flow of lymph fluid, containing the white blood cells – major players in the immune system.

THE LYMPHATIC SYSTEM AND WELLNESS

One of the functions of the lymphatic system is to act as part of a 'sewage system' for the cells. Every cell in your body is surrounded by lymph. You have four times as much lymph fluid in your body as you have blood. Blood is pumped from your heart through your arteries to the tiny porous vessels called capillaries. The blood carries oxygen and nutrients to the capillaries, where they are then diffused into the lymph around the cells. The cells, having intelligence for what they need, absorb the oxygen and nutrients necessary for their health and excrete toxins, some of which go back into the capillaries. Dead cells, blood proteins and other toxic material are removed by the lymph system. Deep breathing and stretching activate this lymph system.

The body's cells depend on the lymph system as the only way to drain off these large amounts of toxic materials and excess fluid, the presence of which can restrict the amount of oxygen available to the cells. The fluid passes through the lymph nodes where dead cells and all other poisons (except blood proteins) are neutralised and destroyed. Many of the 'fight back' cells of the immune system are stored in the lymph nodes. The lymph system is important, because if it were to shut down for twenty-four hours, you would die as a result of blood proteins and excess fluid being trapped around the cells. Think of how a city smells when the bin lorries are not removing rubbish!

The bloodstream has a pump – your heart. However, the lymph system doesn't have one. The way lymph moves is through gravity and physical movement (one of the reasons we turn while we are sleeping). It also is activated by deep diaphragmatic breathing and muscular movement. Think of what you do when you wake up after a snooze? You may stretch, you may yawn, and will often take a deep breath to shake off the feeling of weariness. When you yawn, this moves the diaphragm – a large flap of muscle in the chest. This triggers the movement of lymph and removal of the toxins that accumulated while you were resting. If you want to have a healthy bloodstream with effective lymph drainage and a strong immune system, it is essential to develop the ability to breathe deeply to produce the necessary physical movements that will stimulate action.

Dr. Jack Shields, a highly regarded lymphologist from Santa Barbara California, conducted an interesting study of the immune system. He placed miniature cameras inside people's bodies to see what would stimulate a cleansing of the lymph system. He found that a deep breath from the diaphragm is the best and most effective way, creating something like a vacuum that sucks lymph through the bloodstream and multiplies the pace at which the body eliminates toxins. It has been shown that deep breathing and exercise can accelerate this process by as much as fifteen times!

Dr. Otto Warburg, Nobel Prize-winner, and director of the Max Planck Institute for Cell Physiology, studied the effect of oxygen on cells. He was able to turn healthy cells into malignant cells simply by lowering the amount of oxygen available to them. This research has been replicated many times since.

What does all of this mean to us? Researchers have come to believe that lack of oxygen seems to play a major role in causing cells to become malignant or cancerous. It certainly affects the quality of life of the cells. Dr Andrew Weil suggests, 'Proper breathing nourishes the central nervous system and establishes a harmonious pattern for other bodily rhythms and also regulates moods and emotions'.

Remember that the quality of your health depends on the quality of the life of your cells. Thus, fully oxygenating your system would seem to be a number one priority, and breathing effectively is certainly the place to start. Researchers generally agree that cancer cells hate an oxygen-rich environment!'

One in three people will die from cancer. Athletes experience only one case of cancer to every seven in the general population. Why? The suggestion is that athletes are giving the bloodstream its most important and vital element, oxygen. They are also triggering their bodies' immune systems to work at maximum levels by stimulating the movement of lymph through physical activity. The problem for most of us is that we have never learned how to breathe properly!

There is no one perfect method for breathing. However, if you're planning to respond effectively against illness, here are some methods that have been shown to improve diaphragmatic breathing. Any trained medical person, health coach or yoga teacher will be able to teach you other methods to enhance your breathing and to improve the efficiency of your lymph system.

1:4:2 BREATHING METHOD

1. For a count of ten breaths, breathe in the following ratio: inhale for one count, hold for four counts, and exhale for two counts. So if you inhaled for three seconds, you would hold for twelve seconds and exhale for six seconds.
2. When you exhale for twice as long as you inhale, you eliminate toxins via your lymphatic system. When you hold for four times as long, you can fully oxygenate the blood and stimulate your lymphatic system. When you breathe, you should start from deep in your abdomen.
3. As part of your 'fight back' programme, you might explore repeating the breath work for ten such breaths, in the 1:4:2 ratio, on at least three separate occasions each day. You can even do it sitting in the car or waiting in a queue. It can soon become habitual.

FULL CHEST BREATHING

This approach to breathing effectively is to expand your lung capacity. The two objectives of this method are: to expand the capacity of the lungs and to increase blood oxygen levels. This exercise should be done twice a day and each session should take less than 5 minutes.

Lie comfortably on the flat of your back with the knees bent and the feet close to your buttocks. Take a few moments to 'arrive' and focus on what you are about to do. You are going to concentrate on three separate areas: the belly, the mid-chest, and the upper chest – one stage at a time, mindfully and intentionally.

Belly

1. Resting your hands flat on your stomach with the middle-fingertips meeting at your navel, observe the breath for about a minute without changing it in any way.
2. Now exhale completely and, pursing the lips, exhale any residual air as though blowing out a match. Immediately begin to inhale, but breathing only into the belly (allowing the fingers to part), inflating the belly it as though it were a ball. Do your best to avoid breathing into any other part of the lungs.
3. When you have filled the belly to the maximum, hold the breath for a count of seven.
4. Now exhale gently.
5. When you have exhaled completely, again, pursing the lips, exhale any residual air as though blowing out a match.
6. Hold – with the air completely exhaled for a count of three.
7. Then begin the inhalation process again, breathing only into the belly.
8. Repeat this three times in total.
9. Relax completely and allow a few normal breaths to occur at their own natural pace.

Mid-Chest

1. Now move the hands so they are resting in the middle of the chest and again the middle-fingertips are touching and you can feel the edges of the ribcage under your hands.
2. Now exhale completely and, pursing the lips, exhale any residual air as though blowing out a match. Immediately begin to inhale, but breathing only into the centre of the chest, feeling the ribcage opening up under your hands and the ribs moving away from each other. The upper chest and belly should not be moving too much.
3. When you have filled the mid-chest, and the ribs have opened to the maximum, hold the breath for a count of seven.
4. Then exhale gently.
5. When you have exhaled completely, again, pursing the lips, exhale any residual air.
6. Hold – with the air completely exhaled, for a count of three.
7. Then begin the inhalation process again, breathing only into the mid-chest.

8. Repeat this three times in total.
9. Relax completely again and allow a few breaths to occur at their own natural pace.

Upper-Chest

1. Now move the hands so they are resting on the upper chest and the middle-fingertips are touching approximately at the notch of the collarbone.
2. Exhale completely and, pursing the lips, exhale any residual air as though blowing out a match. Immediately begin to inhale, but breathing only into the upper chest, feeling the top of the chest opening up. Initially, you will find very little capacity here but it will come with time. Do your best to avoid breathing into the mid-chest or belly.
3. When you have filled the upper-chest, hold the breath for a count of seven.
4. Then exhale gently.
5. When you have exhaled completely, again, pursing the lips, exhale any residual air.
6. Hold – with the air completely exhaled for a count of three.
7. Then begin the inhalation process again, breathing only into the upper-chest.
8. Repeat this three times in total.
9. Relax and allow a few breaths to occur at their own natural pace.

Integration

1. Resting the hands back in the mid-chest area, middle-fingertips touching, exhale and begin a partial filling of the belly area, followed by a partial filling of the mid-chest area, followed by a partial filling of the upper chest area.
2. When the lungs are full, hold for a count of seven and allow an exhalation.
3. Repeat this complete breath at least three times, starting in the belly, then moving up to the mid-chest and finally to the upper chest.

   Remember you are seeking to create a balanced, yet complete, breathing habit that ensures full oxygenation of the lungs and blood stream.
4. Always breathe to match your present capability. Do not strain. Remember the maxim of 'passion and gradualness'. If you feel dizzy or light-headed, breathe normally for a while, and then continue in your own time. If all you can do is do a few breaths mindfully today, that's perfect! You've made a good start.

~ SUMMARY ~

When you develop skills in breathing, you are directly improving your immune function.

UNIT 19

NUTRITION, DIET AND FUELLING

Some of the leading dietary causes shown to contribute to, or promote, cancer are excessive fat (particularly rancid, oxidised fat and modified vegetable oils), insufficient fibre intake, several food additives, and inadequate antioxidant and immune system nutrients.

The human body is extremely adaptable. The way we normally eat, when we are in the fullness of health, is challenging enough for the body: rushing meals, not chewing, being absorbed in TV, eating in anger, or sluicing food down with copious amounts of beer, wine, water, tea or soft drinks. As far back as the 1900s, Franz Mayr, a German physician, developed a method of eating that proved to be helpful in assisting the body to detoxify itself, and to make the entire process of digestion less demanding for the physical system.

A person who is 'health-challenged' and who is looking to trigger a healing response in the body will usually benefit enormously from 60–90 days of optimum eating. Before you look at the guidelines, do remember these are guidelines and NOT instructions. They are principles to aim at, knowing the more you can implement these, the greater the effect you will produce.

GUIDELINES FOR OPTIMUM FEEDING OF THE HEALTH-CHALLENGED BODY

How to eat

- Take enough time – at least 30 minutes for each meal.
- Serve foods that are attractive to look at and to eat.
- Eat slowly, in comfort and leisure.
- Take small bites.
- Chew carefully and ensalivate every bite until the food is liquid. Food well chewed is food already part-digested, and so it is metabolised (turned into energy) more easily!
- Savour each bite and eat mindfully. As an experiment, take a single raisin and place it in your mouth mindfully. For about a minute, just roll it

about without chewing it or swallowing it. Muse on the raisin itself, the country it came from, the soil from which it drew nourishment, the sun that shone on it, the rain that gave it moisture, the vine upon which it grew, the workers who tended it and transported it.

Now for about two minutes, actually chew the raisin without swallowing. Under no circumstances swallow until the two minutes are up. Pay close attention to what you experience in your mouth. Have fun!

- You are providing fuel for your body. Free yourself from distractions and disturbances (newspaper, conversation, television, radio etc.) Focus on what you are doing with exquisite attention. Frequent small meals are easier on the body than large ones.
- Ensure that all liquids have been mixed with saliva before swallowing as this aids digestion. This includes water.
- Large volumes of liquids should not be taken with meals, as they tend to dilute the digestive juices in the stomach and add an avoidable 'stress' element. If you want, take small sips of water. In a short time, the body rediscovers the ability to produce saliva.
- If you use dentures, make sure that they fit and that the bite is aligned.

When to Eat

- The body carries out much of its own repair work at night as you sleep. However, it takes 8–12 hours for the bulk of a meal to pass through the digestive system. Your gastrointestinal tract is about 85 metres long! Have you ever noticed how you feel on waking, having had a very heavy meal late the previous night?
- A large proportion of the energy in the food you eat is actually utilised in the process of digestion. Therefore, if you want to make things easy for your body in self-repair, eat your main meal at midday and a light meal in the evening, so that when you lie down to sleep at night, your digestion is essentially finished, and the body can concentrate on repair and renewal.

What to Eat

- Subject to instructions from your physician or nutritionist, you should eat a variety of foods on the basis that a little of what you fancy is good for you. The jury is long since back confirming that that saturated fats and sugars put excess stress on the body. If you want to minimise such stresses during your recovery, you should broadly follow the guidelines of the cancer societies worldwide.

These include:

- Minimising the amount of red meat, dairy produce, processed sugar and saturated fat that you consume.
- Maximising on complex carbohydrates such as wholemeal bread, grains and rice, potatoes and pasta.
- Consuming moderate amounts of fish and a wide variety of fresh fruit, vegetables, pulses and nuts.
- Eating foods as close as possible to their natural state and focusing on 'alive' water-rich foods: carrots, for instance, are better juiced than cooked; green vegetables, the darker the better.
- Consuming foods that have been steamed or gently cooked as they are easier for a health-challenged body to digest than roasted or fried food.
- Frequently, the side-effects of medication will include loss of appetite and constipation – so the temptation might be to skip meals or eat irregularly. Nutritionist Patrick Quillan points out that 40% of cancer patients are mal-nourished. The best way to avoid constipation is to increase dietary fibre in our diet. The faster the food travels through the intestine, the less danger that any carcinogens in the food can adhere to the intestinal lining.

  The best way to ensure a fibre-rich diet is to 'mind your Ps and Qs'. Pears, Peaches and Prunes are an excellent source of dietary fibre, as well as essential vitamins and minerals as is the humble potato. If you want a change from pasta and rice, try Quinoa (available in health stores). It is a mild-flavoured grain, easily digested if you are feeling fragile, and is an excellent source of vitamins and minerals, as well as being abundant in dietary fibre. If your appetite is off, you may find that it is easier to eat small quantities of nourishing tasty food more frequently, than facing the prospect of a normal-sized plateful.
- If you have not traditionally eaten a vegetarian or raw-food diet, a sudden transition to such a diet can be an additional stressor. We recall a patient some years, who, although having a serious advanced cancer, had been in medium-term stable remission. She went to a 'healing centre' where she was encouraged to shift immediately to a raw vegetarian diet. She developed a severe bowel obstruction and died within ten days.

  In making change, be gentle to your body and make the shift gradually.

How much to eat

- The major modern diseases such as cancer and heart disease come partially from stress overload, under-exercising and overfeeding with the wrong foods. It is important to eat regular yet small meals and these meals should match your energy output. Experimental underfed but under-nourished laboratory mice will live twice as long as overfed ones. We have often wondered why patients in hospital are fed such inappropriate foods in quantities that they would need only if they were working on a building site!
- Remember that success depends on consistent adherence! It's what you do daily that counts! If you fail, just climb back on the horse, if necessary with a little support.

~ SUMMARY ~

You are what you eat on a daily basis.

KEY NOTES

'Being involved in the programme helped me to keep focused and committed to actioning behaviour that would help my recovery . . . I also found *Tipping the Scales* was a terrific help and still consult it from time to time, so much so that I have given it to some seriously ill people and their families and recommend it to others.' *J.R., Dublin*

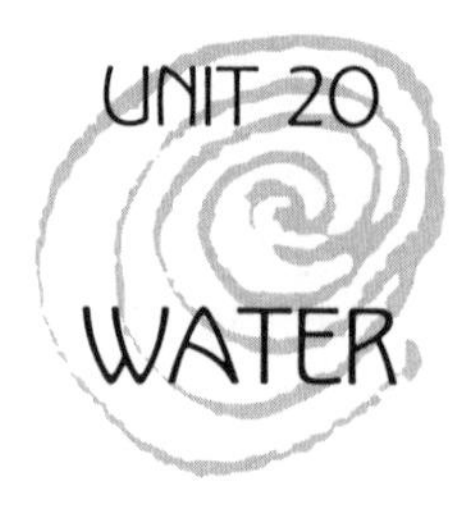

UNIT 20 WATER

People who are ill frequently become dehydrated without even noticing. We lose water through our natural eliminations (faeces and urine) as well as through perspiration and breathing – approximately two pints a day, over all. While taking chemotherapy, potent medications, or perhaps experiencing 'night sweats', the body needs even more water. Lack of water inhibits the immune system.

The environment your cells live in is not blood; it is fluid called lymph. The lymphatic system requires not only oxygen, but also adequate supplies of water to function at its best. Our bodies are 90% composed of water. We can live without food for perhaps 60–90 days, provided we have access to water. Without water, the kidneys pack up, and we die of toxin poisoning in five to ten days. Water helps the body to flush out such toxins and residues from medical treatment. If you don't keep a regular flow of water through the drains at home, what happens? They clog! The human body is no different. Ensalivate all liquids rather than gulping them down; sip rather than sluice! Drink at least eight glasses per day of quality water (filtered or boiled).

Due to chemicals added to urban water supplies and agricultural chemicals leeching into rural systems, it is a worthy investment to purchase an effective water filter. Health food shops are a good source of information on these

Remember that these guidelines are not necessarily for the rest of your life. However, they are essential if you are seeking to offer your body an absolute optimum healing environment.

~ SUMMARY ~

Water keeps your body hydrated and clear of toxins.

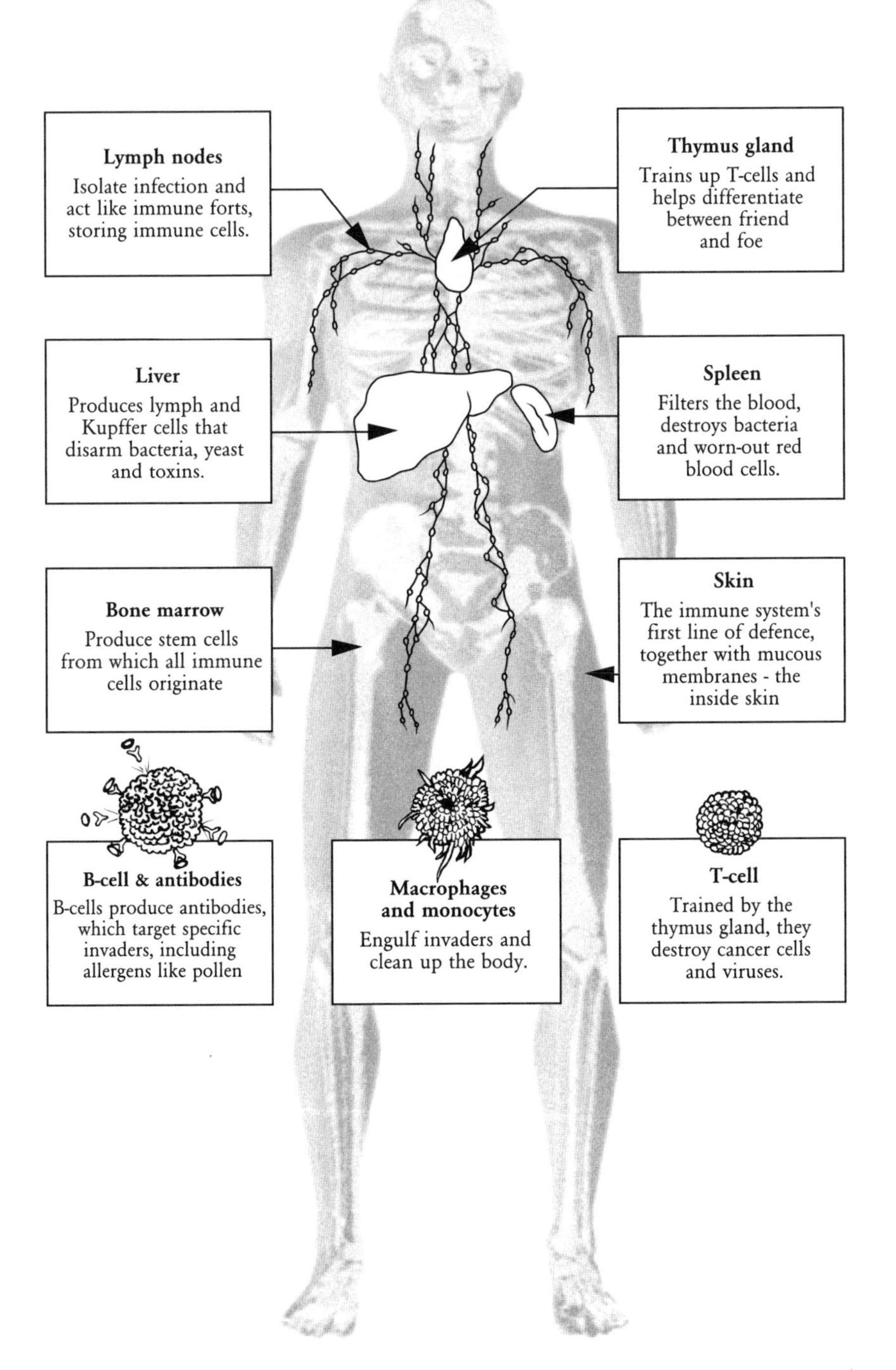
THE IMMUNE SYSTEM
Lymph nodes
Isolate infection and act like immune forts, storing immune cells.
Thymus gland
Trains up T-cells and helps differentiate between friend and foe
Liver
Produces lymph and Kupffer cells that disarm bacteria, yeast and toxins.
Spleen
Filters the blood, destroys bacteria and worn-out red blood cells.
Bone marrow
Produce stem cells from which all immune cells originate
Skin
The immune system's first line of defence, together with mucous membranes - the inside skin
B-cell & antibodies
B-cells produce antibodies, which target specific invaders, including allergens like pollen
Macrophages and monocytes
Engulf invaders and clean up the body.
T-cell
Trained by the thymus gland, they destroy cancer cells and viruses.

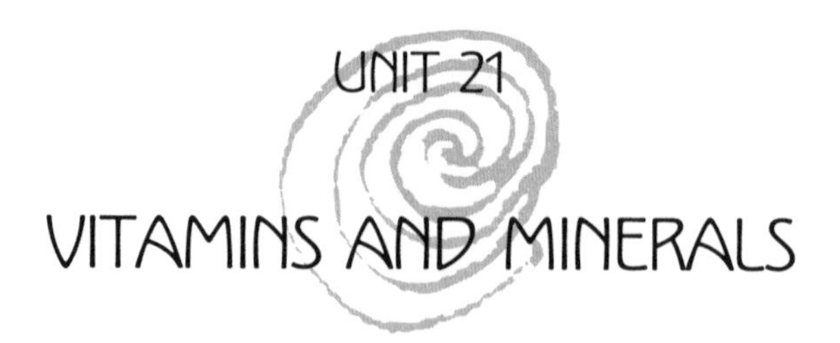

UNIT 21

VITAMINS AND MINERALS

A significant part of offering your body an optimum environment for healing is in making sure your vitamin intake is adequate. Most processed foods are significantly depleted in vitamins. Similarly, many medical treatments result in vitamin/mineral depletion in the body. How do you address this when you may be feeling generally unwell or undergoing treatment with side-effects like nausea, vomiting, etc? The answer is by no means straightforward.

Medical knowledge about nutrition, and in particular about vitamins, remains incomplete, but certain trends are emerging. Patients are often caught in the middle of media hype and controversy. They hear or read about the usefulness of some vitamin or mineral for a certain condition, but when they ask for advice, their doctors often dismiss their questions, saying that there should be an adequate supply in a normal diet.

True, the vitamins coming from eating a varied diet are probably of better quality and do more good than the synthetic variety. However, if you are unable to eat a very good diet, due to your illness, medical treatment, or a food intolerance, then it will do you no harm to take a multivitamin tablet daily. It is wise to check first with your doctor, though it is likely that he or she will advise a moderate amount of vitamins only.

VITAMIN A

Vitamin A deficiency has been shown to correlate with cancer occurrence and progression. However, large doses of vitamin A can be harmful. Vitamin A, found in liver and several other fatty foods, is metabolised in the liver and can cause toxic effects if taken in excess. On the other hand, some vitamins in larger amounts have effects that may make them useful as treatments for particular problems, effects largely ignored by many nutritionists and doctors. It is up to you to explore and find out what might be useful for you!

VITAMIN C

Vitamin C is a popular favourite to take as a supplement. It is needed by the body on a daily basis to aid tissue healing. Its role in the prevention of infections is still controversial, but given that it is harmless, even in large doses (the body easily dumps the excess), if you want to take it, that's fine. Nobel prize winner, Dr. Linus Pauling claimed that 1–3 grams a day of Vitamin C could help to retard the progression of some cancers and, in certain cases, cause them to go into remission. Dr. Andrew Weil describes vitamin C as, 'useful as an antioxidant, cancer fighter, and immune system protector.' The debate goes on.

VITAMIN E

There has been some interesting research on the link between heart disease and vitamin E. A study of a large number of men in Scandinavia showed that those with ischemic (oxygen starvation) heart disease had significantly lower levels of vitamin E in their blood than healthy men. A recent study at Cambridge University of patients with heart disease showed that a supplement of 400 IU of vitamin E each day, reduced the probability of a repeat heart attack by 75%. Vitamin E is found in oily fish and certain other foods, and is known to help lower cholesterol levels. Cancer cells despise the oxygen-rich environment fostered by vitamin E in the bloodstream. Vitamin E has also been shown to potentate or amplify the effect of chemotherapy and inhibit many cancers.

It would seem sensible therefore, if you have cancer, to make sure that you eat oily fish such as salmon, tuna, herring and mackerel on a regular basis. But remember that cooking food in fat destroys over 80% of the vitamin E content. You might consider a supplement of vitamin E, particularly if you dislike oily fish or if you want to make absolutely certain you have an adequate intake. Dr. Andrew Weil describes vitamin E as a powerful and natural antioxidant offering protection against heart attacks and thrombotic strokes – a vitamin which is essentially non-toxic, even in mega-doses.

MINERALS

Mega-doses of most vitamins are automatically dumped by the body if not required. Minerals, on the other hand, are more complex, and it is important to seek medical advice before you consider taking mineral supplements. Be aware that many drugs, including diuretics, can alter the balance of minerals in the blood, and that some cancers may cause a build-up of high levels of calcium, which can make you feel tired, nauseated and unwell.

Reduced levels of magnesium, zinc and other minerals are a rare cause of illness in the general population and unusual even in the presence of serious illness such as cancer. The body needs only tiny amounts of minerals, and usually manages to maintain levels adequately by its own self-regulation processes. However, there is some research to suggest that supplemental selenium can act synergistically with vitamin E to prevent prostate cancer and, to delay progression in those already diagnosed.

BASIC GUIDELINES

Vitamin C	1-3 mgs per day at intervals
Vitamin E	400-1,000 IU per day
Selenium	200 mcgs per day
Co-enzyme Q10	30 mgs per day
Zinc	10 mgs per day

Calcium and mineral levels can be measured by a blood test – you can ask your doctor to include this with your next routine checks.

Supplementation for cancer remains controversial. However a very comprehensive data base of specific vitamin and mineral therapies used in the treatment of cancer (as reported in professional journals) can be found on the Life Extension Foundation website (www.lef.org).

~ SUMMARY ~

Medical treatments tend to deplete vitamins and minerals in the body. It is essential to compensate for this.

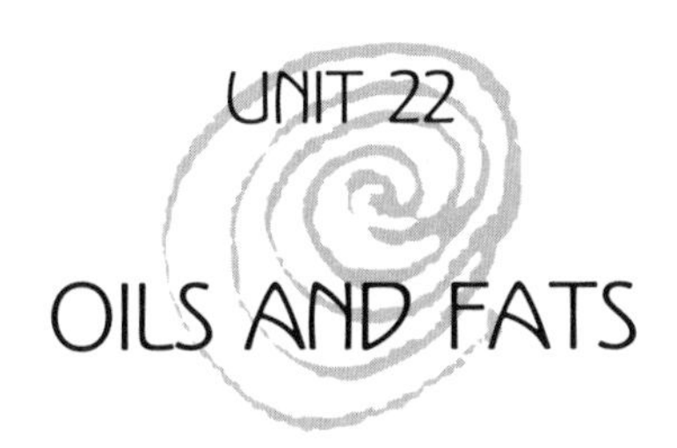

UNIT 22

OILS AND FATS

For many years now we have been reading about the negative effects of saturated fats in our diet. We are encouraged by the main health agencies to eat fruit and vegetables in profusion, a goodly dollop of carbohydrate, oily fish and some protein. The ones that get the green light are polyunsaturated and, more recently, monounsaturated fats.

Although research has long since shown that chemically altered oils and fats are detrimental to health, the consumer has only recently been alerted to that fact. We have been advised to look out for the word 'hydrogenated' on vegetable-based butter substitutes, and to avoid them. We have been told of the dangers of 'trans fatty acids', which are the result of hydrogenation. Although they are difficult, if not impossible, for the body to process, these chemically altered fats are present in almost all pre-packed foods we buy from the supermarket: bread, biscuits, cakes, soups, breakfast cereals, etc.

Very low fat products (including those advertised as 98% fat free) are being promoted as the 'healthy option'. Fat is what makes cooked food taste good – so even without the fat there, no mention is made of the very unhealthy flavour enhancers and refined sugars that are needed to make these products tasty.

Unfortunately, both Eastern and Western cultures are attracted to foods that are fried, roasted, grilled and barbequed. They smell and taste very appetising! Foods cooked at very high temperatures (so that the outside is a tempting dark brown) are potential carcinogens. This is due to the change in the molecular structure of the fats which, in turn, when eaten interferes with the natural function of our cells.

GOOD OILS

What has not been sufficiently emphasised, especially by the health agencies and support organisations, is the fact that certain oils and fats can help boost the immune system. Their anti-oxidant qualities can actually promote the growth of natural killer cells and rid the system of toxins. These are fats that have the right proportion of Omega 3 and Omega 6 amino acids and need to be included in any comprehensive recovery programme.

These fats, in the correct combination, can actually lower cholesterol and, rather than make us fatter, help us to get rid of excess weight! They can help reverse the onset of arthritis and joint pain. They can make our skin smoother and more supple.

A medical doctor on one of our wellness-recovery programmes drew our attention to the book *Fats that Heal, Fats that Kill* by Dr. Udo Erasmus. This book details the negative effects of some oils and fats that are most commonly used in Western kitchens – and also the positive effects of other oils and fats that can actually promote health. He shows that most oils are extracted using heat and this actually changes the chemical compositions of the oil molecules. Apart from the virgin olive oils (green in colour), the other oils, including those advertised as 'high in polyunsaturates', have been refined and deodorised using harsh chemicals. These oils have gone through so many harsh treatments that many of the nutrients and essential fatty acids are removed. The human body does not recognise the molecular structure of these oils – it doesn't know what do with these 'non-self' substances. The result is hardening of the arteries or cancer.

Essential fatty acids are believed by Dr. Udo Erasmus to inhibit tumour growth. Deficiency in these is associated with the occurrence of cancer. He recommends using only pure 'extra virgin' olive oil for cooking. For therapeutic purposes (as described above) cold pressed oils with a 2:1 ratio of Omega 3 to Omega 6 can be taken in a variety of ways, limited only by your imagination. They can be used in salad dressings, added to soups and casseroles (after cooking), fruit smoothies and so on. The blend that he himself developed (using cold pressing) is called *Udo's Choice*, and is widely available in health stores throughout the country.

Dr Barry Sears, author of the *Omega Rx Zone* reports animal research suggesting that high levels of Omega-3 oils can enhance conventional treatment and lower the risk of metastases or spreading of a cancer. However, a considerable amount of research is needed before any firm conclusions can be drawn concerning the effect essential fatty acids/Omega-3 oils may have on cancer.

~ SUMMARY ~

Saturated fats feed tumours and encourage the development of cancers. They need to be eliminated from the diet. Essential fatty acids including Omega 3 are a viable substitute which research suggests may help the body to control cancers.

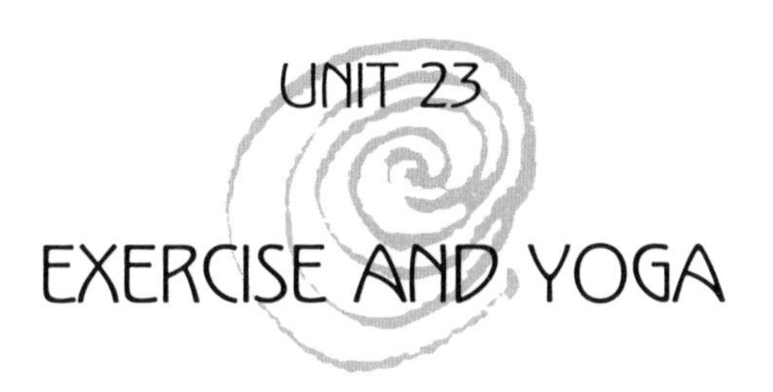

UNIT 23

EXERCISE AND YOGA

Bodies heal less rapidly and less completely when they are not cared for. Dr. Jon Kabat-Zinn, of the University of Massachusetts Medical Centre, describes Hatha Yoga as an ancient discipline of 'gentle stretching and strengthening exercises, done very slowly, with moment-to-moment awareness of breathing and of the sensations that arise as you place your body into various configurations known as postures'. Yoga is available to anyone, and numerous studies are showing it to be a very powerful adjunct to any healing programme.

REASONS FOR PRACTICE

Dr Dean Ornish demonstrated, in 1989, that it is possible to reverse heart disease using yoga, meditation and group work. Dr Jon Kabat-Zinn has been running the stress programme at the University of Massachusetts Medical Centre for more than twenty years, using yoga and meditation as key components. Studies of his work have shown measurable clinical improvements with medical patients with such diverse conditions as heart disease, cancer, lung disease, hypertension (high blood pressure), headaches, chronic pain, seizures, sleep disorders, stress-related digestive problems and skin problems, to name just a few.

Apart from the encouraging clinical medical evidence which is now emerging, yoga as an adjunct to standard medical treatment is attractive because:

- It ensures a gentle massaging of all the internal organs of the body and stimulation of the immune processes.
- It is user friendly and can be practised lying down, sitting in a chair, in a wheelchair or in bed.
- All that needed is that you are breathing and some voluntary movement is possible.
- Any age group can work with yoga.
- It is suitable for virtually all medical conditions.
- It is accessible, with courses available countrywide.
- No prior knowledge, training or fitness capability is needed.
- It is gentle and progressive.

MYTHS

For years, people have been fascinated by images of Indian yogis, twisting their bodies into strange and exotic poses. These adepts will have spent many years training and usually practise yoga for 2–3 hours a day. This has nothing to do with the practice of yoga for therapeutic purposes as part of a 'fight back' programme which involves fifteen to twenty minutes daily of gentle stretching and relaxing.

EFFECTS OF REGULAR YOGA PRACTICE

- Increases mindfulness
- Increases sensitivity or awareness in the body
- Increases flexibility
- Improves sleep patterns
- Stimulates and improves the function of the internal organs and hormonal systems
- Improves metabolism and absorption of nutrients from foods
- Develops breathing and blood oxygen levels
- Encourages healthy lymph function
- Enhances immune function
- Reduces pain
- Increases awareness of eating, food quality and quantity
- Reduces depression and increases sense of well-being

KEY POINTS

You may start at any level of wellness, fitness, or proficiency. If all you can do is lift your hand one inch today, hold it there mindfully, inhaling and exhaling, and then relax it, that is more than enough! You have started on the journey. This is good yoga.

Your objective is to move into a 'posture', hold in that position mindfully for a few seconds, and then release and allow the posture to integrate.

Therapeutic yoga is not about being challenged. It is about 'caressing' or 'kissing the edges of challenge'. Your objective is to stretch into a pose approaching that point of mild challenge, hold mindfully for a count of five and then release.

If you push yourself too far, you will probably either give up or at the very least, retard your progress.

Fifteen to twenty minutes a day is all it takes. If you go to a weekly class, you're more likely to stick with the practice. Also, working with a sociable group actually adds to improving immune function. Your yoga teacher knows what your condition is and what you're seeking to achieve. It's a mistake to be secretive about your condition!

The regular practice of yoga sends an important message to the unconscious mind and to the immune system.

As your health improves, it is tempting to become 'competitive' with other members in the class to prove how much better you are. Forget it! The only person to compete with is you. You stretch towards the edges of discomfort . . . and no further.

GETTING STARTED

The easiest and most useful way to learn yoga is with a trained teacher. Yoga Therapy Ireland or the Irish Yoga Association (or any national association) can provide lists of such teachers. Keep in mind that few, if any, of these teachers are trained to work specifically with medical conditions, but that should not discourage you. Discuss it with your doctor, and advise your yoga teacher about your condition. Ask that teacher to design a specific programme. Most bookshops have excellent beginner's books on the subject.

The illustrations overleaf show a selection of postures that you may care to explore, keeping the above principles in mind. Do remember that an illustration or picture is something to move towards, and is NOT something you have to achieve today. Remember, as we said earlier, if all you can do today is lift one hand mindfully, hold it for a breath or two and then allow it to relax, that's perfect.

Starting today, incorporate fifteen to twenty minutes of gentle stretching (with awareness) into your daily routine. A useful book you might like to look at is *How to Use Yoga, Mira Mehta*, Lorenz Publishing (1994).

~ SUMMARY ~

Yoga stimulates the immune system through stretching and breathing.

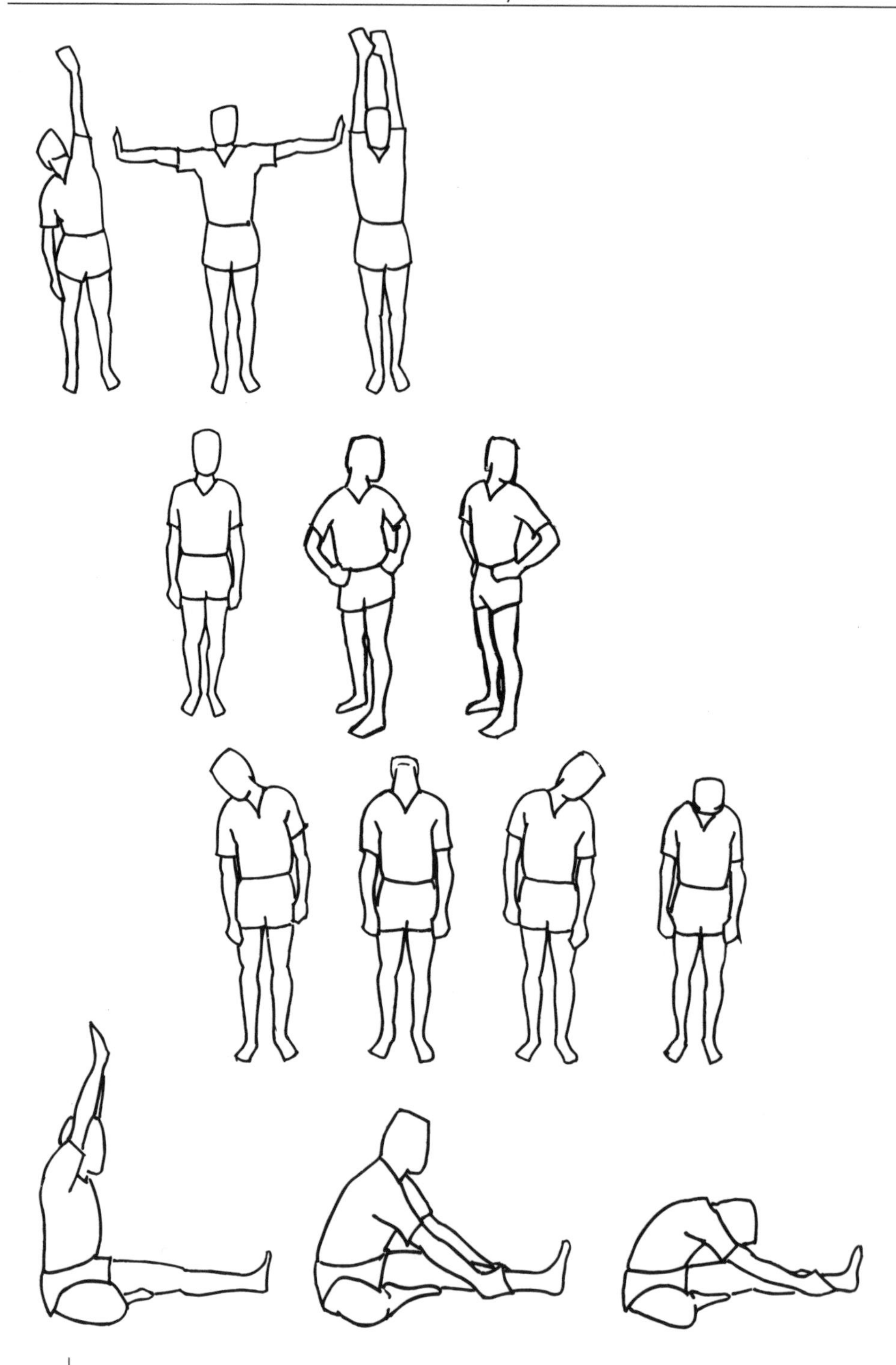

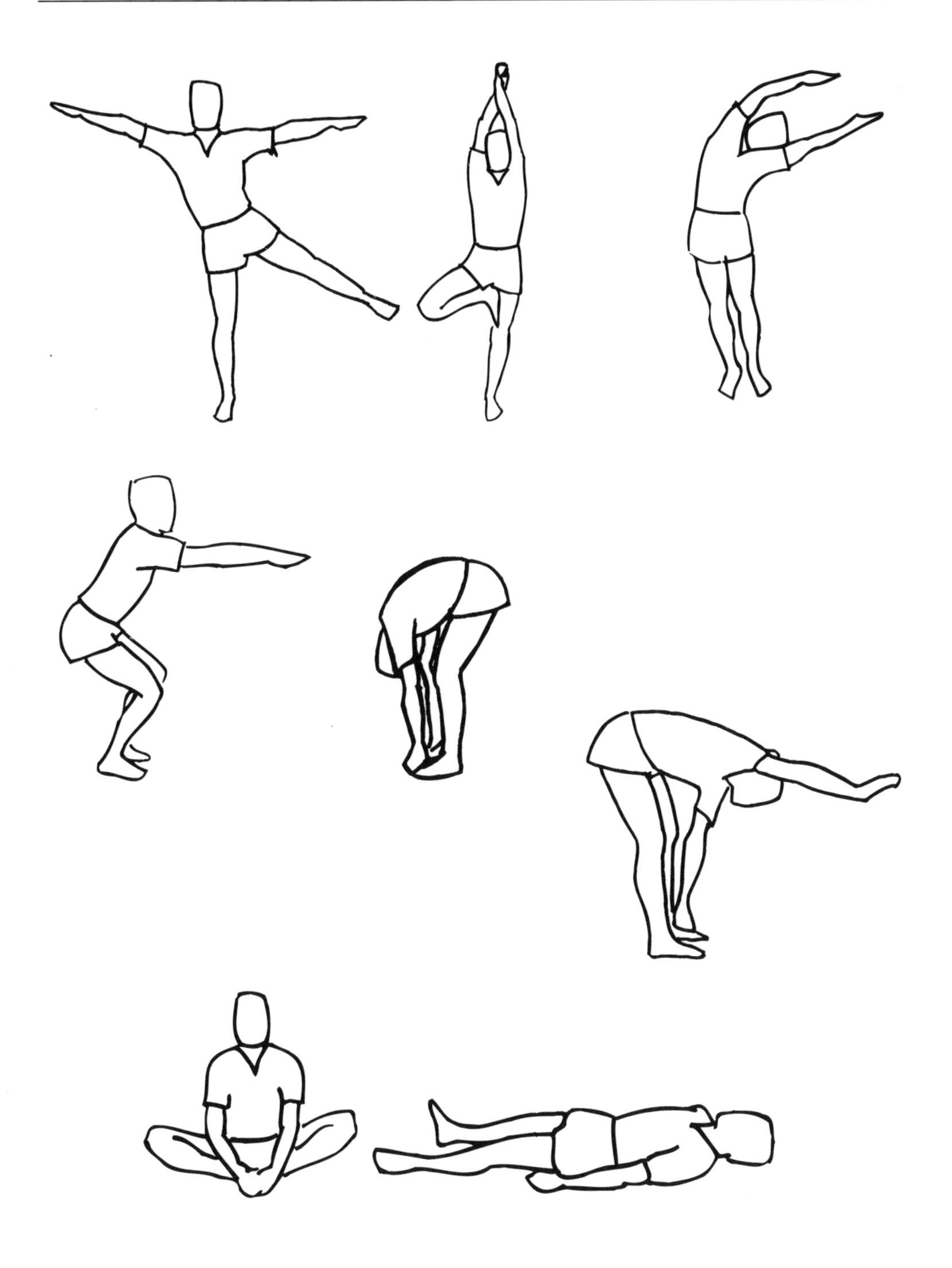

UNIT 24

SLEEP MANAGEMENT AND NAPPING

When a human body is challenged by illness, compounded by the side-effects of medical treatment, it requires more rest and recovery time. This is unfortunately also the time when people experience broken sleep patterns. As mentioned elsewhere, the emotional trauma of diagnosis often adds to this. In addition, as therapists, we are frequently appalled at clients who mistakenly believe that taking sleeping tablets is some sort of admission of failure, or that taking a nap is indicative of 'giving in to the disease'. The reality is that even a healthy body needs six to eight hours sleep a day to repair and rebuild itself. If it is chronically denied this sleep, it becomes ill very quickly. It is, therefore, common sense to offer a health-challenged body even more rest time to heal itself.

A common characteristic identified among survivors of serious cancers is their ability to be 'self-ish' and to take additional time for sleeping. They do not wait for the body to become debilitated or exhausted. They adopt a napping regime early! Researchers often comment on the lower incidence of heart disease and cancer among Mediterranean populations and attribute this not only to diet but also, in part, to the habit of taking a 'siesta' at midday. A 20–30 minute doze has been shown to be effective in allowing the body to recharge its batteries. Here, the animal kingdom also provides a lesson. When animals are sick, they sleep.

SLEEP THOUGHTS

You need more sleep when you are health-challenged. If your sleep pattern is broken, get help in the form of medication, hypnotherapy, self-hypnosis or Thought Field Therapy along with a relaxing bedtime routine.

Naps are invaluable, and can be taken anywhere. All you have to do is become sensitive to the needs of your body. The time to start napping and getting more rest is when you are first diagnosed, not when you are exhausted and run down.

Adopting a different sleeping strategy and addressing sleeping difficulties promptly during recovery is simply putting your shoulder behind your own self-healing mechanism.

SUGGESTIONS

- Take gentle exercise 3–4 hours before sleep.
- Go to bed at approximately the same time each night.
- Avoid going to bed too early.
- Avoid coffee and other stimulants close to sleep time.
- Take a luxuriant bath (not too hot).
- A little aromatic oil, such as lavender, is fine – avoid strong fragrances.
- Gentle breathing exercises help sleep.
- Keep a notebook beside the bed for things you want to remember.
- Use a sleep tape or soft music.
- Practice self-hypnosis for sleep.
- Keep the bedroom for sleep only, not for work projects, etc.
- Keep the room cool and the blankets warm.
- Say 'NO' to television.
- Use an answering machine for the phone.
- Wake up – and get up – at a regular time. Over-sleeping in the morning can trigger a headache!

~ SUMMARY ~

Good sleep patterns and naps help
the body in its response to cancer.

KEY NOTES

PART 3

SPIRITUAL

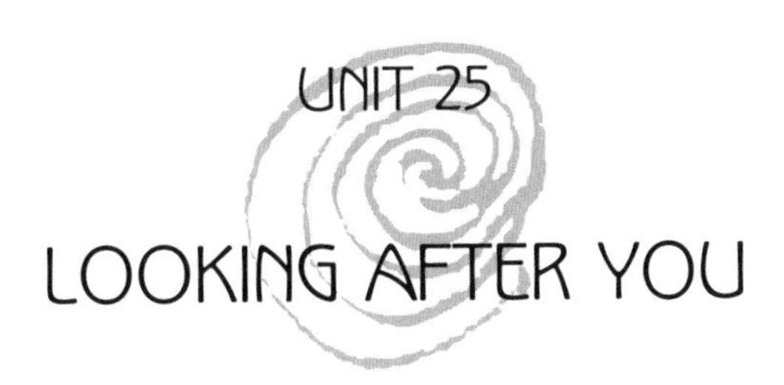

UNIT 25

LOOKING AFTER YOU

We often ask patients what do they really like doing. Invariably we get all sorts of unique responses. We then ask them 'When did you last do these things' or 'How much time do you spend each month doing these things? Invariably the answer is 'Very little!'

Now pose yourself the question: 'When did I last do any of the following?'

Breathe with awareness?
Buy flowers for yourself?
Chat with a friend?
Dance at the crossroads?
Daydream?
Practice yoga?
Do some gardening for fun?
Experience fascination and wonderment?
Go to a concert/play?
Fly a kite?
Paint a picture?
Give money to a tramp?
Ring a long-lost friend
Have an indulgent massage?
Smile spontaneously?
Meditate?
Visit an art gallery?
Read a book/poem?
Sing a song/Listen to music?
Sit and take stock?
Walk in the park?
Spend time with a sick/lonely person?
Take an unplanned weekend away/self-indulgent break?
Spend time in nature?

Is the answer, 'Months' or even, 'Years' to some of the activities? If so, and if there are activities on this list that you really enjoyed – and would still enjoy doing – ask yourself, 'What are the implications for my health if I don't make time to nourish all aspects of myself?'

~ SUMMARY ~

Doing things you enjoy feeds your spirit.
This nudges your body towards wellness.

KEY NOTES

'I learnt a new way of being and a new pace of life.'
A.G., Co. Dublin

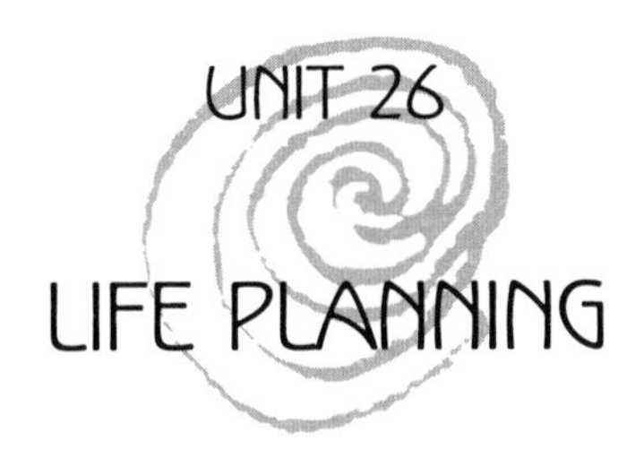

UNIT 26

LIFE PLANNING

If you don't know where you are going,
you will probably end up somewhere else
ANON

In preparing for even a short trip abroad, most people set out a list including such things as where they are going, what they want to see or do and what they will need (passport, tickets, money, clothes, etc.). The vast majority of people however wander through life rarely if ever committing to paper what they really want, and then wonder why they encounter disappointment, or become run-down or ill.

In 1953, a student in a university in the United States found that less than 3% of his class had a written life plan. Twenty years later, another researcher checked with the graduates of this class and found that the 3% with written goals had accumulated more wealth than all of the other 97% together! While only wealth was measured in that study, it suggest proof positive that the unconscious mind delights in and responds to clear direction!

PRINCIPLES OF LIFE PLANNING FOR HEALTH-CHALLENGED PEOPLE

If you have a life-threatening illness, it is probable that your unconscious mind received some sort of negative programming at the moment when you were first diagnosed. Depression and negative emotion weaken immune function. If you want to enhance your immune function, carrying out a review of your life priorities and developing some precise long-term plans for your future tends to let the unconscious mind know that you wish to be around to enjoy them!

The more precise and detailed your plans, the more effectively the unconscious mind will work towards achieving them. Life plans should be reviewed regularly and, if necessary, changed. Clearly defined long-term goals provide the basis for short-term goals and action plans.

THE TEN MOST WONDERFUL THINGS IN MY LIFE RIGHT NOW!

(10 things I would most hate to lose!)

1. ______________________________

2. ______________________________

3. ______________________________

4. ______________________________

5. ______________________________

6. ______________________________

7. ______________________________

8. ______________________________

9. ______________________________

10. ______________________________

THE TEN LEAST WONDERFUL THINGS IN MY LIFE RIGHT NOW!

(10 things I would just love to be rid of!)

1. ______________________________

2. ______________________________

3. ______________________________

4. ______________________________

5. ______________________________

6. ______________________________

7. ______________________________

8. ______________________________

9. ______________________________

10. ______________________________

INVENTORY OF YOUR LIFE – AS IT IS RIGHT NOW

NOW (today's date): ______________________

I am ______________________

____

(*Where are you in terms of career/occupation/job?*)

I own ______________________
(*What do you own or possess that's meaningful to you*)?

I am accomplishing ______________________

____

(*In terms of your personal development, life ambitions, hopes and dreams?*)

I am living ______________________
(*Location in the world?*)

I earn annually ______________________

My net worth is ______________________

My spiritual development is ______________________

____

(*Where are you, now, in terms of evolution of the spiritual or non-material side of yourself?*)

My physical health is ______________________

____

(*What is my activity capability on a scale of 1 to 10?*)

My special relationships are ______________________

____

(What are your special relationships? What sort of shape are they in, on a scale of 1 to 10)?

My hobbies are ______________________

____

(What do you do just for fun or enjoyment? How often?)

My contributing involves ______________________

____

(What do you do for others, in particular, for those who are not family or friends?)

Time ______________________

Money ______________________

Other ______________________

Photocopy and repeat the above section:
(a) dated 20 years from now,
(b) dated 10 years from now,
(c) dated 5 years from now,
(d) dated 1 year from now.
Fill in the answers as you would like them to be.

BACK TO THE FUTURE

The reason for going from the distant future back to now is that it sets a scenario for the 'big picture' of what you see yourself experiencing in life. Working backwards gives you a more accurate idea of the steps or stages that will best take you there. By completing this exercise, you are providing some precise guidance for your own powerful unconscious mind.

ACTION PLAN – TEN THINGS I WILL DO TO PROMOTE MY LIFE PLAN

What are the ten most effective things I can do, during the next 30 days, to get me on my way towards making my life plan real?

1. ______________________________

2. ______________________________

3. ______________________________

4. ______________________________

5. ______________________________

6. ______________________________

7. ______________________________

8. ______________________________

9. ______________________________

10. ______________________________

Remember a plan is only a plan and you are the boss. Just like going on a holiday, you are free to change it and reorganise the priorities at any time.

If you like what you have planned, make a contract with yourself now, in writing, to implement these steps – accepting that you are human, that you may 'fall off the horse', but vowing to just climb back on and develop the necessary skills to be able to do this. Tell someone else what your contract with yourself is. This helps in terms of motivation.

~ SUMMARY ~

Plans pre-programme your unconscious for success. If you don't plan your life, someone else or circumstance will do it for you.

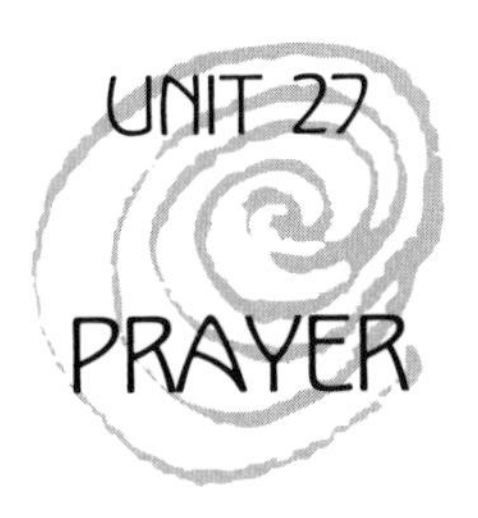

UNIT 27
PRAYER

Clients we have worked with over the years have ranged from being agnostic to having deep faith. On a personal note, I (SC) do remember, when I had a heart attack, that the coronary care unit seemed to have fewer agnostics than one might meet outside in the street. When a person is health-challenged, he is more likely to remember the old maxim, 'In times of trouble, man remembers his God.' The question is however, does prayer actually work?

In 1988, Dr. Randolph Byrd explored the effects of intercessory prayer on heart patients in San Francisco General Hospital's cardiac care unit. His research was a randomised, controlled, double-blind prospective study, involving nearly 400 patients over a six-month period. As patients entered the cardiac care unit, they were randomly allocated to one of two groups. Approximately half of these patients were assigned to Group A to be prayed for by prayer groups of differing denominations up to 300 miles away; the other half were assigned to Group B, which was not remembered in group prayer. For each patient in Group A, five to seven people in various locations prayed for that individual, being aware only of the patient's name and medical condition.

Patients in Group A turned out to be five times less likely to require antibiotics, three and a half times less likely to experience pulmonary oedema than Group B, and none of the prayed-for patients in Groups A needed artificial airways, whereas 6% of Group B needed them.

If you or someone you care about is seeking to tip the balance, to remove 'one straw from the camel's back' so that it's no longer at risk of breaking, then, regardless of your own religious views, can you afford to exclude prayer for self or others from the equation?

~ SUMMARY ~

Even if you do not believe in prayer, you have nothing to lose by having others do it for you. The research suggests there may be a benefit.

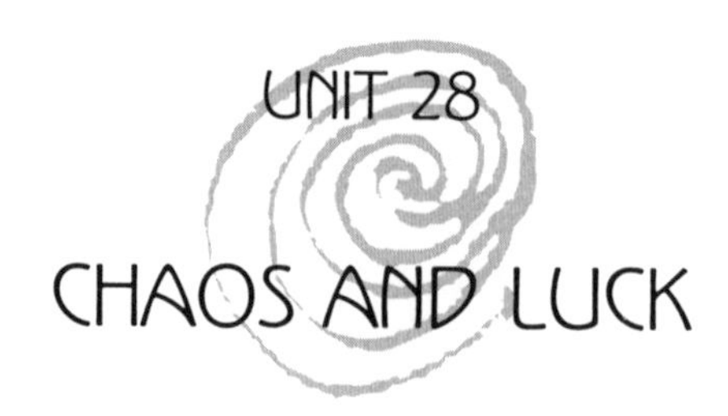

UNIT 28

CHAOS AND LUCK

Something we have observed with research groups is that patients are often nervous of or reluctant to become proactive in their own recovery in case they fail. They see patients around them who do nothing and yet recover. They see others with a 'fight back' attitude who do everything and yet deteriorate and die.

The reality is that behavioural medicine is a little like entering a draw in which 100 tickets are to be put into the drum. Only 99 tickets are available to be bought! If you buy only one ticket, you may win. If you buy 99 tickets, you may still lose. The question is then, how many tickets would you like to have when entering the draw of wellness-recovery. (*See* The Dosage Effect in Behavioural Medicine, page 154.)

The hand of luck is always present in the background of our lives.

~ SUMMARY ~

If you do everything possible, you will have given yourself your best chance for recovery. Even if you still lose the battle, the very least you will have is a sense of having given things your best shot!

KEY NOTES

PART 4

THE 90-DAY PROGRAMME

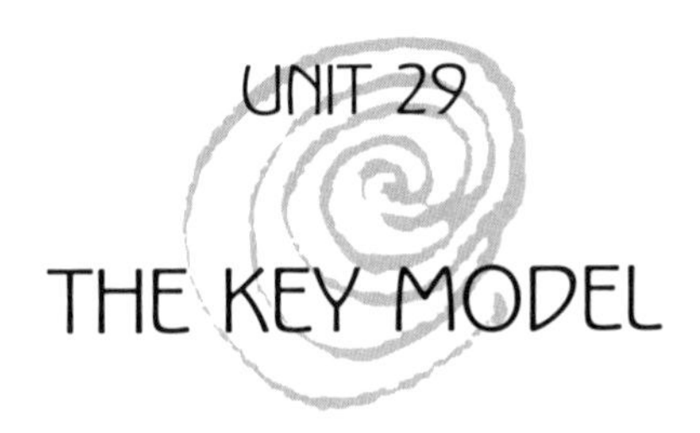

UNIT 29
THE KEY MODEL

A 90-DAY BEHAVIOURAL MEDICINE PROGRAMME FOR CANCER PATIENTS WHO WANT TO FIGHT BACK AND TO HEAL

The following is a 90-day programme in behavioural change. To use an old cliché 'If you keep doing what you've always done, you'll keep getting what you always got. If you want something different, then you'll have to do something different'.

Because many of the soft tissue cells in the body renew themselves over an estimated 90-day period, it is suggested that a successful wellness-recovery programme will need a similar time scale to achieve success. When making a contract with yourself to engage in a structured plan, it is important to recognise that this is not a contract for life. It is simply a contract to act and think in a particular way for 90 days. This offers your body's innate automated self-healing mechanism an optimum environment in which to bring about wellness, something it has been doing all your life.

This programme is designed to help people, both patients and carers, to mobilise their inner psychological resources for taking better care of themselves as a complement to any medical treatment received. The objective is to identify, and then provide an 'optimum' environment in each of the aforementioned areas. As far as possible it is based on 'evidence' from research in the fields of Behavioural Medicine and Psychoneuroimmunology (PNI).

THEMES

Although each week has a specific theme or themes, each builds on the work of the previous one. Like a menu in a restaurant, the programme seeks to offer choices and options. Even if you can engage in only half of the techniques or can only give a 50% commitment, this is fine – for the moment! Numerous studies suggest that more than 85% of participants will produce significant and clinically measurable improvements. You can too! Do remember, if you start this programme, you are committing to an immediate lifestyle change by practising for 1-2 hours a day.

THIS IS WHAT YOU ARE LETTING YOURSELF IN FOR!

Time Commitment 90 days

Daily Projects		**Over 90 days**
Yoga/dynamic stretching	20 mins per day	
Walking	20 mins per day	
Meditation	20 mins per day	
Breath training	10 mins per day	
Self-hypnosis/visualisation	10 mins per day	
Mindful eating	5 mins per day	
Mindful hydration	5 mins per day	
Drug/treatment self-talk	5 mins per day	
TOTAL		143 hrs

PLUS Other Projects		
Life plan (once off)		3 hrs
Well-Formed Outcome/personal contract for 90 days		2 hrs
Un-useful self-talk challenge	0.5 hr per week	7 hrs
Un-useful beliefs/attitude challenge	0.5 hr per week	7 hrs
Support Group	1 hr per week	12 hrs
Counselling/therapy	1 hr per week	12 hrs
Journalling for 5 days in each month	20 mins a day	5 hrs
TOTAL		**48 hrs**
OVERALL TOTAL		**191 hrs**

~ SUMMARY ~

For an investment of a little more than two hours a day over a three-month period, you can dramatically improve your prospects for recovery.

STEPS TO FIGHTING BACK

- Understand your diagnosis.
- Feel and experience what you're feeling.
- Get a second opinion.
- Get a counsellor/mentor/strategist.
- Decide and specify exactly what you want to achieve.
- Go for the best anyone has ever achieved before.
- Explore all possible contributors to your illness and blocks to recovery.
- Explore all possible solution components for your 'fight back' plan.
- Settle on a specific plan and a time scale.
- Explore, and have a strategy for the inevitable setbacks along your chosen path.
- Settle on an evidence procedure for success/failure. How will you know you've succeeded?
- Contract with yourself to follow your plan for a 90-day period and then review.
- Choose a start-date – and begin. Notice what's working and what's not working, and make changes accordingly.
- Keep changing your approach and making adjustments until you achieve the results you want.

THE KEY MODEL PROGRAMME

WEEK 1

- Get an independent second opinion if you have any doubts.
- Read the notes on meditation. If possible get some guidance. Start meditating daily.
- Decide on what to eat and drink, when and how, and start mindful eating (optimum).
- Select a coach/mentor/counsellor and get together with them. Plan for weekly meetings.
- Develop a Well-Formed Outcome for yourself in relation to your health crisis.

WEEK 2

- Find a class/teacher in dynamic stretching or yoga and breath work. Start a daily 20-minute practice.
- Read notes on visualisation and start a daily practice (5 mins twice a day).
- Continue daily meditation.
- Continue daily mindful eating.

WEEK 3

- Review your diet and explore vitamin/mineral supplementation.
- Start self-hypnosis and visualisation.
- Start breath training (5 mins twice a day).
- Start massage/healing therapy.
- Continue daily meditation.
- Continue daily yoga.
- Continue daily mindful eating.

WEEK 4

- Develop a once-off 20-year life plan (3 hrs) and revisit this daily for the week and modify if necessary.
- Continue daily meditation.
- Continue daily yoga.
- Continue daily self-hypnosis and visualisation.
- Continue daily breath training.
- Continue daily mindful eating.

WEEK 5

- Start Laughter Therapy via your support group.
- Start Qi Gong.
- Start challenging Limiting Beliefs.
- Explore Secondary Gain.
- Continue daily meditation.
- Continue daily yoga.
- Continue daily breath training.
- Continue daily self-hypnosis.
- Continue daily visualisation.
- Continue daily mindful eating.

WEEK 6

- Explore Journalling (The Pennebaker Process) to release emotional baggage (20 mins a day for 5 days in each month).
- Use Thought Field Therapy/Time Line Therapy or other psychological intervention, for negative emotion release.
- With your mentor, carry out a review with of all possible causes and solutions to your condition.
- Continue seeking laughter and non-competitive play opportunities.
- Continue daily meditation.
- Continue daily yoga.
- Continue daily breath training.
- Continue daily self-hypnosis and visualisation.
- Continue daily mindful eating.

WEEK 7

- Review Deep Dark Secrets.
- Review your Use of Resources: time, energy, relationships, confidence etc.
- Continue seeking laughter and non-competitive play opportunities.
- Continue daily meditation.
- Continue daily yoga.
- Continue daily breath training.
- Continue daily self-hypnosis.
- Continue daily visualisation.
- Continue daily mindful eating.

WEEK 8

- Again, explore Journalling (The Pennebaker Process) to release emotional baggage.
- Continue seeking laughter and non-competitive play opportunities.
- Continue daily meditation.
- Continue daily yoga.
- Continue daily breath training.
- Continue daily self-hypnosis.
- Continue daily visualisation.
- Continue daily mindful eating.

WEEK 9

- Continue seeking laughter and non-competitive play opportunities.
- Continue daily meditation.
- Continue daily yoga.
- Continue daily breath training.
- Continue daily self-hypnosis.
- Continue daily visualisation.
- Continue daily mindful eating.

WEEK 10

- Again, explore Journalling (The Pennebaker Process) to release emotional baggage.
- Review your 20-year life plan.
- Continue seeking laughter and non-competitive play opportunities.
- Continue daily meditation.
- Continue daily yoga.
- Continue daily breath training.
- Continue daily self-hypnosis.
- Continue daily visualisation.
- Continue daily mindful eating.

WEEK 11

- Review your 20-year life plan.
- Continue seeking laughter and non-competitive play opportunities.
- Continue daily meditation.
- Continue daily yoga.
- Continue daily breath training.
- Continue daily self-hypnosis.
- Continue daily visualisation.
- Continue daily mindful eating.

WEEK 12

- Review your 20-year life plan.
- Review the extent to which you have achieved your outcome.
- Continue seeking laughter and non-competitive play opportunities.
- Continue daily meditation.
- Continue daily yoga.
- Continue daily breath training.
- Continue daily self-hypnosis.
- Continue daily visualisation.
- Continue daily mindful eating.

WEEK 13

- Continue seeking laughter and non-competitive play opportunities.
- Continue daily meditation.
- Continue daily yoga.
- Continue daily breath training.
- Continue daily self-hypnosis.
- Continue daily visualisation.
- Continue daily mindful eating.

RECORDING YOUR DEGREE OF PARTICIPATION

There is a saying that 'what is measured changes'. It has been shown that when patients engaging in Behavioural Medicine recovery programmes as part of a recovery group, maintain daily records of the extent to which they participate in their programme, there is a far greater probability of their persisting to successful conclusion. A clear 'dosage' effect has been demonstrated on many research projects. The more patients engage in the programme, the greater the biological and psychological achievements and consequently the greater their probability of recovery.

Units 30 – 50 contain some of the history and important concepts behind the evolution of the programme. For a health-challenged patient it offers additional background information

PART 5

HISTORY AND IMPORTANT CONCEPTS

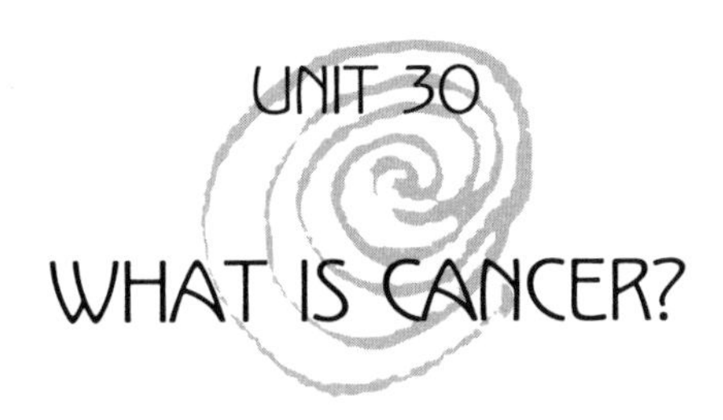

UNIT 30

WHAT IS CANCER?

Cancer is an unfortunate mutation on the magnificent story of the growth of human cells – fertilisation, the division of cells, the transmission of genetic messages from generation to generation, the endless seeds of the human race. In cancer, 'something' happens, probably in the element that regulates all the factors of human growth and the character of cell growth – cell death. Cell multiplication changes, subtly at first, and then with increasing recklessness.

Normal cells, that produce cells with specialised functions, have a life span of just 90-120 days. Cancerous cells, on the other hand, produce 'daughter' cells whose specialised function has been overcome by a powerful, primitive drive for unrestrained proliferation and a hopeless quest after immortality. Fortunately a robust immune system has the capability (not always expressed) to identify these cells and destroy them.

The four major types of cancer are carcinomas (cancer of the skin, glands and organs), sarcomas (cancer of the tissues, bones and muscles), and lymphoma and leukaemia (cancer of the bone marrow/lymphatic/blood system).

Cancer cells, according to surgeon, Sherwin Nuland, 'are spread by the lymphatic system but are generally overwhelmed by the elements of the immune system met along the way, if the lymphatic system is working optimally. Then they will be tackled at a much earlier stage of their development while they are still small'. In other words, they are more likely to succumb to a robust immune response. If not, alteration of cell growth occurs and the cells form colonies of increasing size, eventually becoming detectable by medical testing and diagnosis. Cancer, like most conditions, is a systemic disease.

Cancer is not an acute disease in most cases. It is a chronic disease that takes a long time to be identified with many tumours pre-existing for 8-12 years before detection. The same can be said of atheroma (narrowing of arteries) in heart disease. Many young soldiers killed in Vietnam were discovered, on autopsy, to have significantly blocked arteries, although most men were less than 22 years of age! The stress of being in a war situation was considered to be the major contributor to this blocking!

GROUND BREAKING DISCOVERIES

Professor David Spiegel is a professor of Psychiatry and Behavioural Sciences at Stanford University School of Medicine, one of the leading universities in the world. He is on the editorial boards of eleven medical journals and his research work has been widely published.

In the late 1980s he set out to show that behavioural or psychological interventions could not affect the occurrence or progression of cancer. It is reported that he was frustrated at people for confusing him with Dr. Bernie Siegel (author of *Love, Medicine and Miracles*) because of the similarity in names! Whilst Dr. Siegel and Dr. Carl Simonton (along with others) were making claims for the effectiveness of Behavioural Medicine, there was little hard evidence, at the time, to show that patients could make a significant difference in the progression of their illness.

Professor Spiegel used a study of 86 women with very advanced (Stage 4) metastatic breast cancer. To his surprise, rather than proving that psychological intervention was useless, he found that there had been a doubling of average life expectancy between the intervention group and the control group, and that some of the women from the intervention group were still alive 13 years later! This study has been subjected to rigorous methodological challenges and was published in *Lancet*, October 14th, 1989, and in other major medical journals around the world.

His approach, called 'supportive-expressive group psychotherapy', included exploration of forming strong bonds of mutual support with other patients, facing fears of dying and death directly, re-ordering life priorities, managing relationships with family, friends and physicians, and using hypnosis to control pain, other symptoms and the side-effects of treatment. A similar well-documented study, carried out by Fawzy I. Fawzy, Ph.D., a researcher at UCLA Medical School, showed that participants had better a better immune function, a lower rate of tumour recurrence and a dramatically lower death rate.

Whilst these studies, and others like them, are not the final word on the matter, they provide compelling evidence for exploring such complementary approaches.

Details of Dr. Spiegel's research and program are in *Living Beyond Limits*, Random House Books (1993).

WINNING THE FIGHT AGAINST HEART DISEASE

Until recently, doctors believed that heart disease, the No. 1 killer in Western societies, was irreversible. In 1990, the prestigious medical journal, *Lancet*, published the results of a study carried out by Dr. Dean Ornish, M.D. who, at the time, was head of the Preventive Medicine Research Institute, and a faculty member of the University of California at San Francisco. His research showed conclusively that this belief was no longer supportable.

In his study, Dr. Ornish demonstrated that heart victims could clean out their arteries, provided they had the grit to make radical changes in their lives. One participant said, 'The programme requires a heavy dose of dedication.' Miracles are performed every day in bypass operations, but these arteries frequently close up again; 'Why?' you may ask. Because nothing has been done to address many of the underlying causes, the problem simply reoccurs.

Dr Ornish suggests 14 grams of fat will keep a person going. The average American eats eight times that amount. Many types of fat disrupt the immune system. The body needs good-quality fat, but only a moderate amount. If you are a farmer out in all weathers doing hard physical work, your body needs more fat than normal to run itself. However, if you are a sedantary office worker, you only need a little fat to keep going. There has been quite a debate recently about the best forms of fat to use for optimum health, with some researchers advocating a virtual fat-free diet and others claiming that a balanced amount of protein, carbohydrate and fat is the way to go. A study at the University of Houston explored the effect of diet on patients with pre-existing skin cancer. They found that those who reduced their fat intake from 40% down to 20% developed on average three pre-malignant lesions. Those on the standard fat diet developed on average of ten!

Although 'good' cholesterol is a necessary component in the blood stream, levels of this fat are also negatively affected by diet. They are also negatively affected by stress, particularly chronic stress. Stress-reduction, in the forms of exercise and relaxation training, has been shown to positively affect cholesterol levels.

I (SC) underwent a quintuple (5 graft) bypass in 1997, and never once was I asked the question, 'What do you think contributed to this?' Nobody asked about diet or stress – or anything else.

KEY ASPECTS OF THE ORNISH STUDY

Participants

- Spent an hour a day on yoga and meditation.
- Took a half-hour daily brisk walk.
- Met twice weekly in a group with a psychologist and a doctor.
- Ate a 15% maximum fat diet.

Results of the Ornish Study

- 82% of the participants experienced significant improvement.
- The more a patient engaged with the programme, the more effect he produced (known as a 'dose' effect).
- The average degree of blockage reduced from 61% to 56% (a 17% increase in oxygenated blood flow to the heart muscle!).
- Some completely blocked arteries actually opened!
- 91% reported a drop in heart pain, generally within weeks of starting.
- Angina disappeared in many cases.
- Cholesterol, in many cases, was cut in half.
- HDL, the 'good' cholesterol, increased.
- Severe blockages were the most likely to regress.
- Participants said that without the group support, they could not have kept going in targeting a total lifestyle change, hence the benefit of peer support and group involvement.

Dr. Ornish's work is often ignored, on the basis that it's deemed too hard to persuade patients to engage! We might suggest that this may be a failure on the part of health professionals to equip patients with the support and skills required rather than a valid criticism of the methods used or the results achieved.

Dr. Dean Ornish's Programme for Reversing Heart Disease, Random Century (1990)
This is essential reading for anyone who has heart disease

~ SUMMARY ~

Expressing emotions lengthens life expectancy for cancer patients.

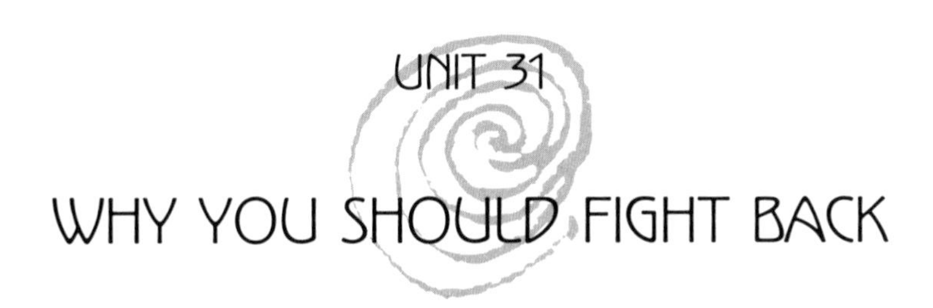

UNIT 31

WHY YOU SHOULD FIGHT BACK

The Key Model is written particularly for those people who want to participate in making a difference. It is not for the faint-hearted. It is for the determined. Ongoing research is showing that patients who proactively participate in their own healthcare have a decided advantage. Frequently a patient, on diagnosis, will ask the doctor, 'What else can I do?' One of our patients quipped, 'Doctors usually have neither the time, the knowledge, nor the inclination to answer this most important question.' While this observation might seem a little harsh, this book seeks to offer a practical response to that question, both for patients and their doctors.

It has fascinated researchers for eons that some seriously ill patients recover completely, while others, with the exact same diagnosis and treatment, do not. As a researcher or patient, I might ask myself the question, 'How come they are so lucky?' We feel however that a much more useful question might be 'How are they doing that?' 'What skills do they have that I can learn?'

Research shows that, at a cellular level, we humans replace all our soft tissue every 90–120 days; our skin every 30 days; our gut cells every few hours; a new liver every six weeks; a new mouth lining every three days; a new skeleton 98% every two years, etc. In other words, you are not the person you were even three months ago – the cells, of which your body is composed, are constantly changing!

Within the DNA and genes of each cell, we carry a specific map or blueprint of perfection that the body uses to rebuild itself. Even when someone has a tumour or a blocked artery, these cells, too, are changing every 90 days. We, as therapists and patients, can use evidence-based methods to restore and assist this blueprint of perfection, and this is where psychological and behavioural approaches are proving useful.

It is estimated that healthy people produce at least 300 potential cancer cells every day, yet a robust immune system identifies any cell that is not normal and eliminates it. When a person is depressed or ill, the immune function is often compromised, leaving space for opportunistic cancer cells to escape detection and establish themselves as potential tumours.

Our objective in writing this book is to load the dice or tip the scales in the direction of optimum recovery by providing the very best possible environment in terms of social interaction, food, emotional state and psychological well-being; also by changing damaging behaviours such as poor eating habits, lack of exercise, smoking, excess alcohol consumption, addictions, depression, short temper, etc. We also need to address so-called chronic negative emotions, such as fear, confusion, or even sheer weariness, which often paralyse the patient and stop him from taking proactive steps to fight back. Greg Anderson of *Cancer Conquerors* says, 'Retaining a medical team without doing all you can do to help yourself is like attempting to walk on one stilt'.

Many doctors, in the course of their everyday practice, see patients engaging in unhealthy or dangerous behaviours. Sometimes they may suggest that a patient drinks less alcohol, stops smoking, eats less harmful fats, eats more fruit and vegetables, takes more exercise, practices stress-management etc. However, mostly they have stopped bothering. It is understandable why many physicians today have become disillusioned about persuading their patients to make lifestyle changes. We, as a society, have fallen into the habit of abdicating responsibility, of thinking that the doctor has a solution for everything, and that we, as patients, have to do nothing. It is no longer disputed that what we eat, how we exercise, how we think and what we do, all combine to make us healthy or sick.

The body often has the wisdom to enclose cancerous cells inside a tumour. When this 'packaging' is perforated during the process of a biopsy, the possibility obviously exists that some cancerous cells may escape into the bloodstream. A single cancer cell, if missed by chemotherapy or the immune system and multiplying on a 90–120 day cycle will take perhaps 6–8 years to become a one-centimetre life-threatening tumour. Therefore our belief is that after successfully overcoming cancer, the immune system needs to be boosted by ongoing engagement in Behavioural Medicine to help the body identify and eliminate any escaped rogue cells. Although we have lots of information on five-year survivals, we do not hear a lot about the frequency of recurrences many years later. Cancer is opportunistic but then so also is health! There is no point in closing most of the windows – and still being burgled! You have to close all the windows.

~ SUMMARY ~

If you don't take charge of your own recovery – who will?

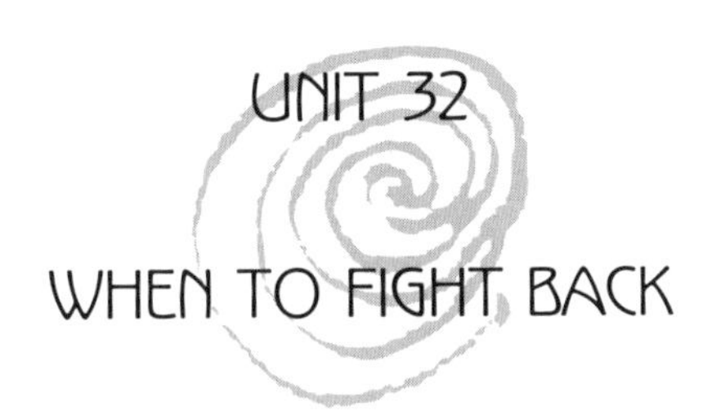

UNIT 32

WHEN TO FIGHT BACK

Let's say that you were asked to take a group of ordinary citizens for a demanding one-week climbing expedition high in the Himalayas. Would you put them on a plane tomorrow with lots of mountain-climbing gear? Or perhaps might you instead consider a preparatory training course? What would you want them to do on this training course? You would obviously want them to acquire knowledge about the conditions they would encounter: weather, altitude, terrain etc. You would also want them to engage in a physical and psychological training course so as to get them into the best condition: developing stamina, robustness and fitness for the challenges facing them.

What then of the misfortunate ordinary citizens diagnosed with cancer or some other life-threatening or 'quality-of-life'-threatening condition. Previously, they had been living an ordinary life, probably were not in peak physical or psychological condition and suddenly they are assaulted by terrifying news. They are catapulted into a frightening world of symptoms, tests, strange words, consultants, treatments and side effects along with potential loss of hopes and dreams.

Unlike our Himalayan group, they receive no psychological or physical training, no preparation, and little or no information. They are just 'put on the plane'. Some will survive; many will not.

The military trains its soldiers for maximum fitness, stamina and adaptability. We believe patients also have a need to develop maximum fitness, stamina and adaptability for their new environment of being a patient. Yet few receive such training: the lucky ones adapt to the medical environment; the unlucky ones don't.

Physical illnesses such as cancer and heart disease are not 'germ-based'. They have been evolving over many years before reaching critical mass, being identified via symptoms and then diagnosed. The average breast tumour is estimated to be 8–12 years old before being found. As mentioned, a single malignant cell, doubling every 90–120 days will, if missed by the immune system, take about eight years to become a one-centimetre tumour if left to its own devices! Once cells become malignant, the process accelerates.

In many cases, diseases such as cancer can be described as chronic rather than acute. In other words, they are moving slowly but inexorably towards the point where they will threaten the host body. Do they need acute treatment like someone who is having a heart attack? In most cases they don't. Can they be neglected? The answer again is 'No'. Is there a window of opportunity for the patient to get into the best possible physical and psychological shape for their surgical/medical 'trip to the Himalayas'? The answer here is 'Yes'! However, because of the current bias in medical thinking, such approaches are rarely if ever suggested to patients, let alone implemented.

Research suggests that you can produce meaningful clinical changes at virtually any stage in the progression of a disease. It takes approximately 60–90 days to get a person into top physical and emotional shape. However, many patients wait until a disease has become well established and aggressive treatment has been implemented before contemplating 'fighting back'. The immune system is our in-built 'fight back' or protection system, the following points are perhaps worth considering.

We know from clinical research that:

- The shock of diagnosis or 'bad news' lowers immune function.
- Chronic negative states such as depression, helplessness, hopelessness, powerlessness, which often follow diagnosis, lower immune function.
- Medical treatments (chemotherapy, surgery, medication, radiation) are powerful assaults on the body-mind. They challenge the body and often lower immune function.
- The sense of social isolation, common to many ill people, lowers immune function.
- The disease and treatment may stop normal physical activity necessary for maintaining or enhancing immune function.
- The disease may interfere with breathing patterns – lowering immune function.
- The disease may cause irregular or broken sleep patterns, which again can lower immune function.
- The actual ongoing progression of a disease frequently lowers immune function due to tumour loading.
- A quirk of human nature is that feeling upset often causes people to engage in potentially self-destructive and damaging behaviours, including increased alcohol consumption, smoking, overworking, etc – lowering immune function.

All the above situations tend to happening at the very time when you would want your immune function to be at its most effective! Any medical programme that concentrates solely on the disease, and neglects consideration of a specific strategy to address the above reactions, is potentially deficient.

Due to financial and time pressures on the medical system, many people today (except, perhaps, the very wealthy) endure months of waiting before being assessed, tested or treated. During this time, intense feelings such as fear and anxiety can trigger the release of damaging hormones which suppress immune function. This waiting time offers a window of opportunity to get yourself into optimum physical and emotional shape in preparation for treatment.

I (SC) have often asked myself, even when people are physically in hospital, either as out-patients waiting for tests, or as in-patients, for what proportion of that time are they actual undergoing medical tests or treatments? The answer is probably less than 10%. The rest of this time is often spent just hanging about, waiting. However that time again offers a valuable opportunity for actively exploring some of the concepts and methods described in this book!

NEW DANGERS IN THE HOSPITAL

Now, if you are planning admission to hospital for surgery you may get more than you bargained for, and it might kill you! In the last few years you will have heard news reports on 'superbugs', one of the most common being MRSA (Methicillin Resistant *Staphylococcus Aureus*). Some of the most virulent of these bacteria are resistant to the most powerful antibiotic, vancomycin, sometimes known as the 'last line of defence'. The reason for this ever-increasing danger is the reckless over-prescription of antibiotics for common winter infections, and from the failure of patients to complete their prescribed courses of medication.

The new trend for using antibiotic soaps and household cleaners is also having the opposite effect of what was intended by their developers. These products are helping to create tougher and more vicious bacteria than the ones normally found on your hands or worktops.

A large proportion of normally healthy mortals carry MRSA strains without any signs or symptoms of illness. However to the frail and elderly, or those with a suppressed immune system due to surgery or cancer treatment, these bacteria can be lethal. According to a BBC report, up to 5,000 patients a year die in the UK due to infections caught in hospitals.

'Why are you attempting to scare me if there's nothing I can do?' I hear you ask. The very reason we are bringing this to your notice is that there are many evidence-based things you can do to raise your immunity and avoid such potentially lethal infections. If you have just been diagnosed with cancer or heart disease, then engaging in a Behavioural Medicine programme as described in this book can be part of your armoury against opportunistic infection. Every single element in the programme adds to your immune potential.

~ SUMMARY ~

If at all possible, you need to start your wellness-recovery programme before commencing conventional cancer care.

KEY NOTES

'Knowing I had choices regarding how I would live with my illness gave me much needed hope. I was to set goals for a future I didn't believe in; that exercise turned despair around. Having to imagine where I would be five years ahead made the possibility that I could be alive real. It's a life-saving programme.' *C.W., Dublin*

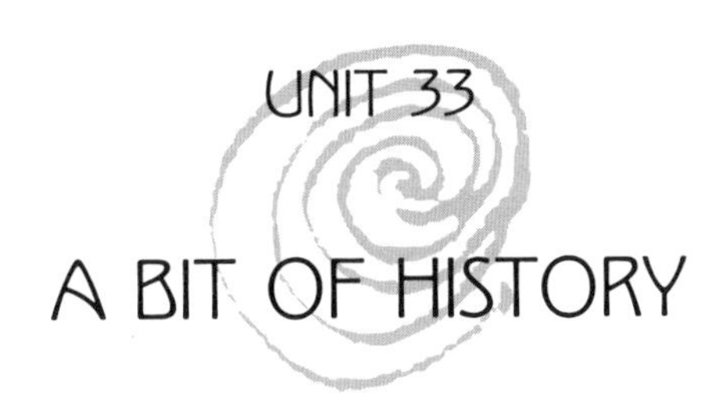

UNIT 33

A BIT OF HISTORY

In the 17th century philosopher and mathematician, René Descartes, formalised the dualistic views of the church into a reductionistic and mechanistic biology. He promoted an approach that left the soul (and thus behaviour and thought) to God, and moved medical investigation of health and illness into a purely secular realm, free of the threats of mentalist or religious considerations. He put forward the idea that body and mind are separate entities. It has been suggested that in order to secure cadavers for autopsy, he and his colleagues entered into an unwritten arrangement with the then very powerful and influential Church, that they could have the mind and spirit if he and his colleagues could have the body for autopsy and research. The emphasis of medicine then shifted to treatment of symptoms, syndromes (groups of symptoms) and dysfunctions of physical organ systems.

In the 20th century, medicine and scientific breakthroughs permitted dramatic advances in the curing of acute disease following on the emergence of the germ theory of disease in the middle of the 19th century. Doctors/scientists took advantage of the scientific method to identify individual sources of disease and illness, and evolved treatments through surgery, medication, vaccination and other new technologies. The stage was set for an accelerated drift away from an integrative bio-psycho-social perspective towards the 'reductionistic' mechanical model. Disease, once again, became just a breakdown in the machine, and it was the physician's job to fix the machine. Doctors stopped viewing the patient as a complete entity or as a vital element in his own treatment. It was left to philosophers to continue to ponder if the mind could influence the body!

Louis Pasteur was best known for his contribution to the original germ theory of disease. However, later in life he is quoted as saying that if he were to undertake new studies of disease, he would direct his efforts towards environmental conditions and varying host resistance. He pointed out that even with bacteria, these could cause damage only when the body is weakened.

The medical model, for the past 150 years, has tended to focus exclusively on the body and what is measurable. According to scientific thinking, 'If its not measurable, it doesn't exist'. However all patients lead as much a psychological and spiritual experience as they do a physical one. Are these measurable? Each patient will respond to the onset of the disease out of his own biological AND emotional and psychological history. Why then are the mind, emotions and soul still substantially excluded from a treatment plan? Surely this is relevant to you as a patient seeking to improve the odds of a complete recovery?

There is no patient whose condition progresses identically or whose condition responds in exactly the same way to treatment as another patient. There is not even a single disease called cancer. There are about 250 diseases which share common elements but which are gathered under the banner of cancer. Norman Cousins, pioneer in Laughter Therapy stated: 'There is no terminal illness known to man that has killed 100% of the people diagnosed with it'.

If you look at a statistical bell-curve of survival in terminal illness: some people die soon, some survive the expected 'normal' time and some defy the odds, gaining entry to the 'winners circle' and live out a full lifespan and/or blow the condition out. With new knowledge, where can you, the patient, aspire to get to on such a survival curve?

Science has tended to regard exceptional survivor patients as 'outliers' (1-5%) and exclude them from statistical analysis in case they might skew the data. Spontaneous remissions and unexpected disappearances of disease confuse science as there is no obvious mechanism, and so they are often factored out as part of 'good science'. However, these survivors offer potential seeds of discovery of a new element in reversing a disease process. We have, in our office, a large tome listing thousands of cases of spontaneous remissions of the most virulent and advanced cancers – all published in peer-reviewed journals. What these case studies do not reveal is what these patients were doing, behaviourally and psychologically, towards recovery. Whether you are a patient or a doctor, it seems reasonable to ask, 'How did these exceptional people achieve remission or recovery if they received the same medical treatment, what is the difference that *made* the difference? What delivered them into the 'winners circle'?

Some research suggests that, without medical intervention, the statistical odds of a complete miracle remission in a potentially terminal condition are slim. When you introduce medicine, you begin to change those odds dramatically to perhaps 2:1. When you consider then adding-in comprehensive psycho-behavioural interventions, might we now begin to aspire towards achieving that elusive full remission for the majority of patients? Current research would strongly suggest that we should.

In the late 1970s, advances in exploring and understanding the immune system revealed a number of ground-breaking studies showing that psychosocial intervention and behavioural change could positively influence immune function and sometimes actually lengthen life expectancy for certain terminal cancer sufferers. Cardiologist Dean Ornish also demonstrated similar programmes that enabled people with advanced heart disease to open and clear their own blocked arteries, something previously considered as medical heresy.

These studies should suggest to you, the patient, that how you think, react and behave will have a significant influence on how well you respond to conventional medical treatment, how well you manage the illness and whether you are likely to achieve a remission, a cure, or at the very least, a significant improvement in the quality of your life.

A real and valid fear has existed among doctors that such findings might prove dangerous to patients. They worry that news of these discoveries might encourage patients to reject conventional treatment. They are also concerned that patients might regard the findings as scientific 'proof' that psychotherapy and other alternative approaches might offer a viable alternative cure for their disease, and might put themselves at risk by turning away from the more difficult avenues of traditional treatment, such as surgery, medication or chemotherapy, and radiation. We concur entirely with this concern. However, suppose you have a healthy shrub in your garden that has been thriving. Then, one day you move it to a shadier and perhaps damper part of the garden where it starts to do poorly. You can prune it; you can add chemicals; you can clear weeds – but are you addressing the real issue? The problem is that the plant has been deprived of its previous 'optimum' environment and is now in a less favourable one. Your measures may be helpful in some conditions, but the real solution for that plant is to restore it to its optimum environment so that it can begin to thrive again. This is what psychosocial behavioural medicine is about – identifying and crafting an optimum physical AND emotional and psychological environment where healing can occur.

To our knowledge, there has never been, in the annals of medicine, a doctor or physician who has ever been evaluated scientifically as having 'healed' anyone. Doctors are the custodians of hundreds of years of good science and medical research. They are highly trained individuals with comprehensive knowledge of illness, disease, treatments and side effects. They have the necessary skills to diagnose and to prescribe treatment yet, in reality, they are providing an optimum environment in which the body's own natural healing mechanisms can operate freely. For instance: if you injure your arm in an accident, the doctor may have the arm X-rayed, he will have the wound cleaned, he will set the bones, he may apply antiseptics and antibiotics, he will have a bandage and splint placed over the injury, but he himself will not do the actual healing. The healing response lies within the individual and not with the doctor.

Surgeon Sherwin Nuland comments, 'As doctors, we do our best when we remove the obstacles to healing and encourage organs themselves to use their own nature-given power to overcome the disease.' Even from a Christian standpoint, I doubt that a just God would elect to heal only those who could afford an air ticket to Lourdes. This healing mechanism comes hardwired into every human body, a blessing of nature and perhaps of God.

In setting out to research this book, it felt like finding pieces of a jigsaw on the road, in no particular order, and without knowing the final picture. From the pieces available, we could only guess at it and then start to look for the corner pieces, the edge pieces, the bits with red on them, the bits with blue on them, the bits with lines, and so on. Anyone who has ever done a jigsaw will identify with how frustrating this can be.

Over the past fifteen years, I (SC) have reviewed more than one thousand books, both technical and popular, along with countless research papers in the area of Behavioural Medicine and discovered that virtually all who achieved a 'miracle cure' or spontaneous remission from cancer, heart disease or other significant condition, had also used the very best of what modern medicine could offer. To our knowledge, there is no evidence whatsoever to support the exclusive use of 'alternative' therapies. What we offer here are evidenced, research-based, methods of providing an effective adjunct to mainstream medical wisdom and not an alternative.

As clinicians and researchers, one tries to look for single factors or groups of factors responsible for an observed outcome. However, working with health-challenged patients, we are allowed to speculate on incomplete evidence and look for useful interventions, providing we follow the old medical maxim, 'First, do no harm!' Virtually everything offered here in *The Key Model* has emerged from solid research at major universities around the world.

It is, of course, important that theories in Behavioural Medicine be put to the test before being accepted into general usage. However, we are convinced that – if reasonable suggestive evidence exists for a technique or approach, if it is certain that it cannot harm the patient, if it creates neither 'false hope' nor 'false despair', if it is done with the knowledge of the patient's doctor, if it does not put the patient at risk of exploitation – patients then must have the option of making up their own minds and join with their medical team in working towards a complete recovery.

I (SC) was prompted to write the predecessor to this book, *Tipping the Scales*, in 1997 because, when I faced a health crisis of my own, there didn't seem to be a straightforward guide on how to be proactive and effective in improving my chances of recovery. *The Key Model* is a second attempt at providing such a tool for patients and for the health professionals working with them. It is far from complete. We doubt any book will ever be complete, as new discoveries in the field of Behavioural Medicine emerge all the time.

Now that national health-care programmes around the world are running out of money, waiting times for treatment are lengthening, and as a society we are dealing with an increasingly ageing population, can health-care providers afford to delay in supporting Behavioural Medicine programmes? Blue Shield Health, one of the world's largest insurers, is now sponsoring research in such programmes with Dr. Carl Simonton. Professor Herbert Benson and Margaret Caudill, at Harvard University, demonstrated a 15% cost reduction by introducing Behavioural Medicine programmes. We, in Ireland, spend in excess of 8 billion on health services. What are the potential savings from Behavioural Medicine, and how might these be used? Just recently, I (RD) heard a leading executive from one of our two major health insurers stating on radio that preventive medicine would be far too costly to cover. Regular screening, X-rays, scans and blood tests, he assessed, would add greatly to the cost of health insurance (rather than saving them a fortune in long-stay hospital charges). The area of psychoneuroimmunology as preventative medicine was even further from his mind. Even from an economic standpoint, Behavioural Medicine saves money!

In a similar vein, we have been asked why doctors do not regularly encourage patients to engage in Behavioural Medicine programmes. The answer seems to lie in the fact that there is little awareness among them about the positive research, albeit fragmented, which has been done. A survey of GPs in Leinster, carried out in 1997, showed that 25% of them had not even heard of Psychoneuroimmunology.

It also seems to come down to money. In expectation of future profits, multinational drug companies will invest vast amounts of money into research on drugs for which they may gain a profitable patent. However, if someone develops a successful protocol or programme in Behavioural Medicine, the process becomes available to all, and is therefore not commercially attractive.

In academia, the same applies. Academics, researchers and departments in universities are funded by government grants and by industry. Two summers ago, I (SC) met a German research scientist at a traditional music session in West Cork. He asked me what I did for a living. I told him I was involved in research in applied Psychoneuroimmunology or Behavioural Medicine. His cryptic response was 'That has ATF or anti-tenure factor!' In other words, it is an area that does not attract research funds or academic effort!

We all have heard of those who fight back – the so-called 'positive thinkers'.

However, in the real world, we have seen patients who are 'fighters' succumb and die prematurely and seen other patients with negative attitudes thrive and survive. Does this mean that attitude makes no difference? No it does not. Will following a Behavioural Medicine programme guarantee success? No it won't! What it will do is substantially change the odds of success.

At present, few cancer patients are offered a comprehensive Behavioural Medicine programme let alone individual elements. However, oncologist Professor Tim Oliver, of the Royal London Hospital suggests, 'Optimism brainwashing adds 1–10% to the chances of recovery. Not a large percentage, but in many cases, that's all that chemotherapy does!' Professor Herbert Benson of Harvard University has proposed that 'psycho-social intervention should be implemented immediately upon diagnosis/prognosis rather than as a last ditch effort late in the progression of an illness when recovery prospects are materially compromised'.

The Key Model seeks to answer the question: What can the individual patient do to increase the odds of getting into that elusive 'winners circle'? What are the magic ingredients which, when added to the awesome power of conventional medical treatment, can enable a patient to change the odds and live longer and better than all the rest?

Sport researchers study winners and success. Business researchers do the same. The secret in achieving excellence in anything is in studying the successes and also learning from the failures. Regrettably, medicine has tended to study illness, disease and pathology and missed out on the study of the miracle of health and wellness.

'Healing,' said the poet W.H. Auden, 'is not a science but the intuitive art of wooing Nature.'

~ SUMMARY ~

The research is there to support the use of applied Behavioural Medicine.
It can dramatically tip the scales for you
in the direction of full recovery.

UNIT 34

PSYCHONEUROIMMUNOLOGY (PNI)

Psychoneuroimmunology began over 20 years ago with the work of Dr. Robert Ader, who demonstrated that the immune system had the capacity to learn and to be conditioned. Researchers at leading universities around the world have continued exploring how psychological and behavioural approaches might potentially improve immune response. What has emerged – like the many pieces of a jigsaw – are individual studies showing that some psychological and behavioural aspects can contribute negatively to disease and others significantly enhance immune response and recovery prospects. However, not all patients respond to intervention in the same way, and these exciting results have tended to languish in the realms of academic curiosities.

MEASURABLE POSITIVE CLINICAL RESULTS ACHIEVED INCLUDE

- Serum cortisol dropping (enhanced immune function).
- Increased natural killer cell numbers and activity (cytotoxicity).
- Increased numbers of helper-T cells (better immune function).
- Immunoglobulin A (IgA) up.
- Lowered biological body age.
- Normalized cholesterol and blood pressure.
- Improved lymphatic function.
- Improved psychological well-being and vitality.
- Oxygen uptake increase.
- Body fat decrease.
- Less pain and, intriguingly.
- Sometimes longer survival times.

The tests for scientific credibility are: measurability, predictability and reproducibility – all of which have been met!

Modern medicine offers the accumulated knowledge of hundreds of years of good science. However, since Descartes, the mind and its potential impact on health and recovery have been all but neglected. Galileo postulated: 'What cannot be measured and quantified is not scientific' (soon to become bastardised into 'What cannot be quantified is not real!') Although the fields of Behavioural Medicine and Psychoneuroimmunology are still in their infancy (less than 25 years), we suggest they now potentially offer the 'difference' that can *make* the difference.

Researchers Drs. Elmer and Alyce Green, in the United States, examined 400 cases of spontaneous remission. The common feature they found was that all these people had changed their mental and emotional attitude prior to remission and had, in some way, found hope and become more positive in their approach to the disease.

Dr. Dean Ornish demonstrated that the progression of certain types of heart disease could actually be reversed using similar psychological and behavioural methods.

Professor David Spiegel at Stanford showed that life expectancy could be doubled with (Stage 4) metastatic breast cancer through group psychotherapy and self-hypnosis.

Behavioural Medicine is both a process and an adopted lifestyle. What it offers is a respite zone to enable recalibrating of the entire body/mind system and the creating of a buffer for stress.

~ SUMMARY ~

Behavioural medicine has been shown to produce miracles when an optimum environment is provided.

UNIT 35

THE HUMAN RESPONSE TO DIAGNOSIS

So you have been diagnosed with a serious condition. You have been assaulted by news that threatens your future.

We hear a lot about the physical symptoms of disease and the side effects of treatment. We hear very little about the negative psychological and spiritual effects of disease and treatment and, more importantly, their implications for recovery. The response of someone who has just learned that they have a life-threatening or 'quality-of-life'-threatening disease will be complex, and will depend on their own personality and coping style. Later in this book, we describe in detail the body's complex stress response to the combination of the disease, the treatment and the psychological issues attaching to them. More importantly, we present some of the implications of these response mechanisms and their relevance to recovery.

COMMON RESPONSES TO CATASTROPHIC NEWS OR TO A MAJOR LOSS INCLUDE

- Shock
- Disorganisation
- Denial
- Repression
- Anger
- Bargaining/Negotiation
- Depression
- Guilt
- Blaming
- Anxiety
- Helplessness/Hopelessness
- Confusion
- Obsessive Thinking
- Aggression

The question is, 'Are these responses good or bad. Are they useful or not useful? Are they potentially dangerous?' According to traditional psychology, these responses are followed by:

- Resolution
- Acceptance
- Adaptation
- Re-integration.

MOVING FORWARD/SETTING UP ANEW

Theoretical models are not people. Individuals respond in their own unique way, at their own unique pace. Different people may experience all or some of the above repsonses, and in different sequences. Let us examine some of these, and their relevance to recovery.

SHOCK

Shock is a protective state to enable us to adapt or cope with the unimaginable, the unthinkable. If you see someone after a bad traffic accident or a sudden death, you see shock. Shock is like a state of suspended animation where time seems to stand still and the person is numb, feels nothing. It is similar to the 'freeze' response in animals. However, as described later, in a state of shock, a person is highly susceptible to accepting suggestions – either positive or negative – from themselves or others (particularly significant others), which will impact on the condition.

CONFUSION

A person who is shocked will generally experience confusion and disorganisation. They enter a place of chaos where 'what could be taken for granted yesterday is not the same today'. The hormonal response to shock can interfere with the ability to even think straight. What can you trust? Can you even trust your own judgement? Understanding that this is a normal part of our adaptive response can be helpful in the midst of such inner chaos.

DENIAL

Another element in our tool-kit of adaptive responses is denial. When we deny a problem, it reduces or eliminates the shock or confusion so we can attempt to think clearly. US President Bill Clinton was asked how did he felt when questioned in front of other world leaders about his affair with Monica Lewinski. His reply was, 'I compartmentalise.' In other words, he could temporarily deny the prospect of potential disgrace and leave himself able to deal effectively with world affairs.

Heart patients who use denial are often at increased risk in not responding to body symptoms. However, this trait, when carried into the time after a heart attack, has been shown in studies to be useful in that there is less anxiety and more certainty of recovery. In other words, it is paradoxical and can be both a blessing and a curse. However, denial can be risky as we can defer tests or treatment, or even begin to engage in 'unhealthy' or self-abusive behaviours in an attempt to 'prove' that we are well.

ANGER

Prior to diagnosis, we can assume a typical patient has been doing his best to lead a good life. When disease strikes and when all that he took for granted appears to have been snatched away, it seems reasonable for him to ask, 'Why me?' and experience a sense of being angry at the world, parents, children, the Universe, God.

Anger normally lets us know when our boundaries, our values or beliefs have been abused. However, it is also a powerful emotion, potentially spurring us to action. Sometimes it can be referred to as 'blind' as it can block our ability to think clearly. This response, which is sometimes expressed as aggression, can be a challenge for a patient's family or medical carers but must be recognised for what it is – an attempt to exert some sense of personal control in the face of the apparently uncontrollable or irrevocable.

BARGAINING/NEGOTIATION

Even though it makes no logical sense, when catastrophe arrives, we often go into inner places where we attempt to negotiate with the Universe or God. 'If you make this go away, I'll be a better person, etc.' Irrational as it may appear, this again is part of normal adaptation, of coming to terms with catastrophe, of seeking to negotiate a return to where we were.

On hearing of the sudden death of my brother, Michael, in 1990, I (SC) remember the first words I was shouting were, 'Please, don't let this be true!' Who was I talking to? What was the point? But we do it anyway.

DEPRESSION

Depression is another of our strategies for dealing with terrible things. As a short-term state, it is adaptive. We retreat into our cave where nothing or nobody can touch us. Some theorists believe that if we did not become depressed in the face of catastrophe, we would be at greater risk of taking our own lives. Depression becomes like a scab on a flesh wound to allow healing to occur. Chronic or ongoing depression, however, has been shown to suppress the immune system, (our first line of defence in coping with illness or infection) and interfere with our 'fight back' response.

GUILT/BLAMING

Once the reality of diagnosis and prognosis has sunk in and treatment has started, patients sometimes enter a place of guilt or blaming: 'If only I had done more… If only I had done X and had not done Y!' It's all my fault!' They may also go into: 'My mother, father, employer etc. were unjust to me. It's all their fault.'

It is virtually impossible for someone not to have been a part-contributor to most disease processes. While it is natural, sometimes, to seek someone to blame, most conditions are multi-factorial in origin. Guilt or blaming can be part of a healthy transition to a new reality but if the emotion becomes stuck it can become toxic, poisoning relationships, or even, as research suggests, it can contribute to an accelerated disease process.

HELPLESSNESS/HOPELESSNESS

Helplessness means a sense that there is nothing YOU can do. Hopelessness is a sense that there is nothing ANYBODY can do. In the short term, this is normal. If it becomes long-term, this is unhealthy. Researchers such as Professor Lydia Temoshok (formerly of the World Health Organisation) quotes evidence suggesting that these feelings can accelerate a disease process and weaken the body's immune response.

OBSESSIVE THINKING

In 1989 when I (SC) had my first heart attack at the age of 38, I became obsessed with it. My first thought each morning was about my heart and my chances for survival. My last thought at night was, 'Will I survive until morning?' Later on in 1998, on learning of the death of my son, Hugh, it filled all my waking thoughts, it was my last thought before sleep and my first thought on waking. This continued for perhaps eighteen months after his death. However, in that case I was coming to terms with something that was irretrievable. There was nothing I could do to influence what had happened. In the case of the heart attack however, I could begin to acquire knowledge and develop strategies to assist my recovery.

This obsessive-type thinking is useful in a health crisis as it can enable you to focus your energies towards a solution. It is important, however, to differentiate between things that we can exert some influence over, and those we cannot. In the case of a death, there is nothing we can do but learn to live with it. In the case of a disease, there is much we can do.

~ SUMMARY ~

All the above reactions are normal healthy adaptive responses to a catastrophe. However, if they become ongoing and remain unaddressed, research suggests they may contribute to suppressing your immune response, destroy your quality of life, and inhibit your compliance with medical treatment and prospects for recovery.

KEY NOTES

UNIT 36

SELF-HEALING MECHANISM

It is said that we are what we eat, how we exercise, our thoughts, our reactions, our history, how we breathe, the water we drink, our genes, etc. Most of the modern degenerative diseases such as cancer, heart disease, arthritis and diabetes are said to come from our modern 'civilised' lifestyle of over-eating, under exercising, consumption of contaminated foods and environmental toxins.

A phenomenon of the human body-mind system is the amount of abuse it can take. For years, we can avoid exercise, undergo chronic stress, eat dreadful diets – and yet the body-mind hangs in there and tolerates it. Herein lies the risk. This type of overload on the system might be compared to an archer pulling back on a bow. At first the resilience and flexibility inherent in the bow allows you to continue pulling the arrow back. However, there is a point where there is no more give left in the system and if pulled farther, the bow will break. Once it has broken, it cannot be unbroken.

Almost everybody has this automatic self-healing mechanism (SHM). Everyday we are exposed to countless bacteria, viruses and possible infections. We catch a flu virus: the body takes a few days to identify the intruder and work out the right prescription in its own chemist shop and, *voila*, it's gone! Dr Andrew Weil suggests, 'It is a misnomer to call medicine the healing art. The healing art is the secret of the body. Medicine can do no more than facilitate it!'

The living body, as has already been said, is a process rather than an event. It replicates itself constantly. If you vacuum house dust, you find much of it to be particles of dead skin or cellular matter. The question then arises, if the body is constantly replacing itself, why then do tumours continue to exist? Why do scars persist after a cut on your hand?

What has happened is that the replication blueprint in the 'damaged' cells has been altered, so their 'children' are altered as well. Tumours continue to exist and grow. Scar tissue gets formed after a cut. If you have ever seen the scar one month after an operation, it is essentially healed, but is still rough looking and maybe inflamed. However, if you look at that same scar three years (many generations of cells) later, you can see how the inbuilt seeking of a cell to return towards normality has been in action and the scar has faded considerably.

One of the characteristics of cancer cells is that they have lost the in-built message that they are supposed to live ninety 90–120 days, to pass on their genetic messages to subsequent generations and then die. This is how many tumours occur. Collections of cells refuse to die, and try to achieve immortality. However, paradoxically, cancer cells are weaker than normal cells and hence the usefulness of chemotherapy and a healthy robust immune system.

Here is where we have the opportunity to harness the body's own ability to recover, provided the best opportunity is offered. It is often said that your body is a reflection of the degree of balance in your life. Even under the inevitable assaults of drug therapy, surgery and radiotherapy, the body's bounce-back capability comes to the fore and tolerates the treatments, in most cases. Our job in Behavioural Medicine is to add the weight of our shoulder to the wheel and do whatever is possible during a 90–120 day window of opportunity (the average life of a healthy cell) to help the body heal itself through an optimum environment.

When a patient receives treatment to specifically suppress immune function, as is sometimes necessary, does the patient develop all sorts of cancers? The answer is generally 'No', at least not at the time. Somehow, the wisdom of the body figures out ways to keep the system in check! Standard medical treatment for cancer will typically include surgery, chemotherapy and radiotherapy to address the acute or current situation. These all have some negative side effects but they are the best available option. However, what is done about the patient's psychological response to the cancer or the predisposing circumstances or behaviours that may have contributed to it? What is done to stimulate immune function? If anything, standard treatment may well weaken or compromise immune function!

How about the heart patient? Again, standard treatment will initially address the acute symptoms. There may be surgery, a bypass, rest and rehabilitation. There may be drug therapy to bring down cholesterol levels or blood pressure. But rarely is the questioned asked: 'What factors in this person's lifestyle and make-up may have contributed to this incident?' The possibilities may be: heredity, poor diet, smoking, lack of exercise, stress, etc., but when the patient leaves hospital, (frequently with this question unaddressed) he is on his own. He may visit his doctor to have cholesterol and blood pressure taken. The medication may be applied. He may be told, 'Cut down on the fat, take exercise'. But what if the demands of his life take over again? The medication will probably stabilise the situation and suppress the symptoms or warnings, but if his lifestyle doesn't change, then he will probably be back, perhaps even with a fatal heart attack next time. Statistics show that after five years, 40% of heart bypass grafts are partially blocked again. After ten years, failure rates are in the region of 75%.

Another factor seldom addressed is the psychological side effects of long-term medication. Consider that in the case of younger male cardiac patients, drugs to lower blood-pressure can also significantly lower libido and sexual function. This can have a significant effect, not only on the physical aspects of a relationship, but also, most particularly, on self-image. Even if the medication is stopped, the pattern or learned behaviour persists. This frequently results in depression – which, in turn, lowers immune function.

Modern conventional (allopathic) medicine performs miracles in terms of stabilising and keeping patients alive. Early detection surpasses medical treatment every time. However, if the core causes are ignored, if the patient keeps behaving and thinking the way he always has, he will almost certainly arrive back at the same place.

There is an old story of the monk who is walking by a river one day and hears a shout for help. He sees a person drowning in the river and so jumps in and rescues him. As the monk sits dripping on the river bank, he hears another shout for help. Again, he has to jump in and pull another person out. As the monk is catching his breath the second time, he hears yet another shout for help from the river. Once more he is back into the water and pulling another person out. Finally, dripping and exhausted, the monk says to himself: 'I'd better go up the river and see who is throwing these people in.'

In this old story, there is a powerful message for both the medical profession and for governments. The World Health Organisation Charter defined health as 'a state of complete physical and spiritual well-being and not merely the absence of disease or infirmity'. If we do not address in a comprehensive way the root causes of many of these common diseases then health budgets will continue to soar and people will suffer and die unnecessarily.

~ SUMMARY ~

The body and mind know how to heal themselves
if the blocks are removed.

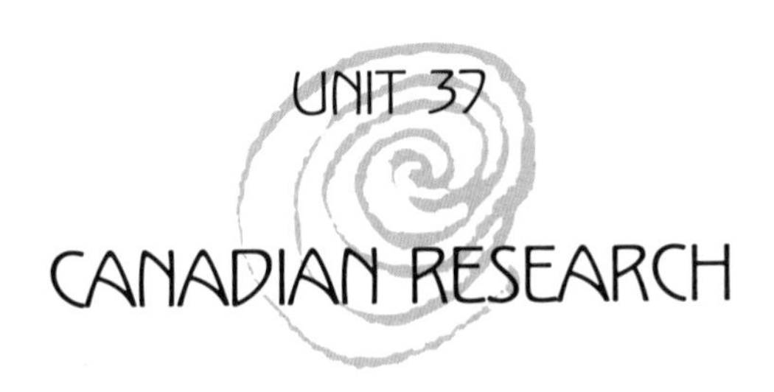

UNIT 37

CANADIAN RESEARCH

In the late 1970s, Dr. Hans Selye, the father of modern stress research and Dr. Richard Earle, the director of the Canadian Institute of Stress, noted that there was a major gap in the existing research on the relationship between stress, health and ageing. We have known for many years that too much stress is damaging but, paradoxically, too little stress (stimulation or challenge) is equally bad both for infants and adults. Dr. Earle designed a research programme to investigate the relationships between these factors, by testing various existing stress-management techniques for their effectiveness in enhancing immune function and lowering body age in healthy volunteers.

Of the 1,868 who volunteered for his study, 623 were selected who tested as having a body age significantly higher than their calendar age. Excluded from the programme were those in current medical treatment for any chronic physical disorder, or anyone in psychotherapy or on ongoing medication. After assessment, volunteers were trained in ten stress-management and anti-ageing interventions.

A comprehensive programme was designed for each individual that related specifically to his unique needs as revealed by psychological testing. Each participant undertook to follow this programme for eight months, and to keep a daily diary of his experiences.

STRESS-MANAGEMENT AND ANTI-AGEING INTERVENTIONS

1. Self-hypnosis and anti-ageing imagery
2. Nutrition
3. Values/goals clarification (career and leisure)
4. Relaxation
5. Physical conditioning (exercise)
6. Cognitive reappraisal (rethinking high-stress situations)
7. Personal goal setting and motivation
8. Communication and conflict resolution
9. Managing decisions, priorities and time.
10. Budgeting 'stress energy'

The results achieved were nothing short of remarkable! After just eight months, they had achieved the following results:

Average body age decreased by	8 years
Doctor visits decreased by	53%*
Days missed at work dropped by	58%*
Below target blood pressure	91%
Weight within 10% of normal	86%
Cholesterol within target range	74%
Immunoglobulin A (IgA) increase	31%*
T cells increase	28%*
Triglycerides within target range	61%
Stress hyper-reactivity down	46%*
Stress recovery time down	36%*
Ability to relax at will increase	31%*
Physical strength increase	39%*
Body flexibility increase	32%*
Percentage body fat decrease	36%*
Oxygen uptake increase	47%*
Forced expiratory volume increase	27%*

(**Note**: all figures are averages and asterisked items show the average improvement of the study group expressed as percentage changes from average baseline scores.)

During this programme, the participants increased immune function by about 30% (T cells and IgA). They enhanced their ability to take in and use oxygen by 35%, indirectly increasing the efficiency of their lymphatic systems. They took eight years off their body age and all of these people were 'healthy'. Current research suggests that patients with cancer, heart disease and other significant health problems can produce even greater results.

For some patients, any one complementary therapy may well be the difference that *makes* the difference. However, individually such therapies cannot predictably reverse any disease process. Let us assume however that any can produce miracle results in, maybe, 5% of patients. What will happen if you apply twenty such therapies or interventions in a Behavioural Medicine programme? The multiplier, or synergistic effect, might suggest that you can more than double the odds of successful recovery.

~ SUMMARY ~

Combining Behavioural Medicine approaches produces a synergistic or multiplier effect.

KEY NOTES

'I was sceptical embarking on the programme, but am now an advocate having completed it . . . The programme gave me techniques to look at my stressors from different perspectives and took me through a number of options and methods of successfully dealing with them.' *C.H., Co. Dublin.*

UNIT 38

DOSAGE EFFECT IN BEHAVIOURAL MEDICINE

It hardly needs saying that the more you do towards taking charge of your own wellness and illness, the better the results will be. We have noticed through our research programmes that individuals who undertook most of the items on the menu of possible interventions, and practised them regularly, achieved much better results than those who simply dabbled in one or two as the spirit moved them! The message here is, 'If you are seeking to change the odds towards full recovery, you need to be whole-hearted about it!' This 'dosage' effect has been noted in numerous international studies.

~ SUMMARY ~

The more you do in Behavioural Medicine,
the more effect you achieve.

KEY NOTES

'The course has given me a confidence which, up to the time of my illness, I lacked.' *O.C., Sligo*

UNIT 39

UNDIAGNOSED POST TRAUMATIC STRESS DISORDER

Many people today will have heard of a condition called Post Traumatic Stress Disorder (PTSD) and its association with Vietnam veterans. Patients suffering with PTSD describe reliving some past traumatic event, experiencing nightmares and flashbacks, difficulty in sleeping, feeling detached and estranged, to the extent that these factors materially impair their lives. By coincidence, many cancer and heart patients describe similar happenings following diagnosis.

Emotions described by patients with PTSD include: fear, panic, helplessness, hopelessness, self-blame, guilt and shame. Problems also arise in relationships, losing interest in things the person normally derives pleasure from such as sex, hobbies etc. Symptoms also include anxiety, hostility, depression, palpitations etc. Longer-term responses include 'shutting down' or feeling emotionally numb. People with PTSD tend to have abnormal, and sometimes chaotic, levels of the key hormones involved in response to stress. They feel out of control. What are the implications of hormonal chaos? Chronic hormonal chaos negatively affects immune function. Just as it has been accepted that many people in society experience undiagnosed depression, equally, many cancer and heart patients find themselves inside a confusing world of undiagnosed PTSD.

Various 'brief' therapy models have emerged in the past twenty years such as Eye Movement Desensitisation and Reprocessing (EMDR), Time Line Therapy and Thought Field Therapy. The discovery of these new brief therapeutic approaches emerged, essentially, from research with patients suffering with PTSD. As time has gone on, these have proved highly successful in resolving chronically stuck emotional states such as anxiety, panic attacks or depression, and in restoring hormonal balance. As an external intervention, they can enable a patient to 'break out' of an unhelpful stuck emotional state. It's tough enough dealing with the illness without loading chronic negative emotions on top.

In our work with cancer patients, we often ask ourselves the question, 'What could be more stressful for a person than the sudden and unexpected diagnosis of a disease which may take their life or, at least, dramatically reduce the quality or length of it?' What of the fact that it may expose them to potentially painful, disfiguring and/or toxic treatment, which may take away hopes, dreams or independence?' When people believe their failures are due to some unchangeable personal deficit, they often lose hope and stop trying. The same applies to patients dealing with a serious disease. The solution may come from a basic belief that setbacks and failures are due to chance circumstances, they are a 'challenge' and you can change them for the better – a belief that can lead to optimism.

For any of us, in everyday life, what are the implications of the ending of a significant relationship, the loss of a career, the death of a loved one, even the process of ageing? PTSD does not affect all patients exposed to a given significant negative life situation. Some will respond to it as a challenge or an opportunity to rearrange their lives. Others interpret it as God's will. Others just give up. We are fascinated to note that virtually nowhere in the literature on PTSD is there any significant mention made of its potential for negatively affecting people encountering serious illness.

How an individual reacts to a negative life situation will depend on many things including their physical condition, age, general health, life experiences, expectations, their natural ability to deal with stress, and the kind of help and support they get from family, friends and professionals. A person diagnosed with HIV or AIDS automatically is assumed to be in need of skilled counselling. Why not so for patients dealing with the bad news of a serious diagnosis or prognosis?

Not everybody who experiences the trauma of serious diagnosis/prognosis will go on to develop full-blown PTSD. Those most likely to be affected will include people who are experiencing the greatest and most intense sense of unpredictability, loss of control, victimisation (real or perceived) and betrayal by God, life, their bodies or the medical system. They will also include those with prior vulnerability factors such as genetics, previous life trauma, lack of social support and concurrent stressful life events. In addition, those with habituated responses of guilt, shame, stigmatisation or self-hate will be much at risk.

An exciting aspect of addressing 'stuck' negative emotion is that there is much that patients can do. Successful intervention can happen either at the physical or psychological level. For instance, a novel approach for treating chronically depressed patients is aerobics. This seems to help the body reset itself hormonally. One reason that exercise is recommended for general health and energy is that muscle activity actually increases the number of mitochondria in cells. Mitochondria are the energy factories of the cell, which turn glucose (the basic fuel of the cell) into the energy-rich substance called ATP. This ATP is the basic currency of energy-exchange in most metabolic processes of life and in virtually all responses to stress.

Lack of exercise has been shown to be involved in high blood pressure, heart disease, diabetes, obesity, osteoporosis, colon cancer, depression, and falls and fractures in the elderly – yet one in five adults is obese. One in three heart attacks or strokes is due to inactivity. Less than 37% of men and 25% of women walk briskly for 30 minutes 5 times a week.

Cardiologist, Dr Dean Ornish, and behavioural psychologist, Dr Jon Kabat-Zinn, have both demonstrated yoga and meditation as highly successful approaches in restoring states of balance to patients suffering with both physical and psychological issues.

If you are a patient who can identify with the symptoms of PTSD described here, then it is likely your defences and self-healing capabilities are compromised. The Pennebaker Process of journalling (*See* page 47), when applied to the moment of diagnosis, is a possibility for correcting this.

~ SUMMARY ~

Undiagnosed Post Traumatic Stress Disorder
can weaken your defences.

KEY NOTES

'I felt I had been given a tool and shown how to use it, a tool I never knew existed before, which was exactly the tool I had been searching for and needed.' *M.G., Co. Dublin*

UNIT 40

VOODOO DEATH AND THE WAND OF THE MAGICIAN

'In the land of the sick, emotions reign supreme;
fear is just a thought away'
SEAN COLLINS

What is a belief? We all have them. A belief is simply a sense of certainty about something. It is a fact that what you focus on expands – what a person believes deeply tends to come true. Can a person's beliefs kill them? Is it possible that doctors and consultants may inadvertently contribute to installing unhelpful beliefs? Is this significant?

Dr. Walter Cannon, the acknowledged discoverer of the human fight/flight response, believed so. To further his theories, he visited countries such as Haiti, New Zealand, Australia, The Caribbean and Africa to study the phenomenon of 'voodoo death'. He found that if a person had the witch doctor's 'bone' pointed at him and he believed he was going to die, in most cases he would die in spite of the very best efforts of medical personnel and medical practice – yet with no pathology existing!

CERTAIN CRITERIA WHICH HAD TO BE PRESENT FOR 'UNTREATABLE DEATH' TO OCCUR (AS IDENTIFIED BY DR. CANNON)

The person had to:

- Receive significant negative information or indirect signs or symbols from a 'prestige' person (e.g. the witch doctor).
- Have a high degree of suggestibility (not gullibility).
- Develop a high degree of negative belief and expectation concerning the pronouncements or actions of the 'prestige' person.
- Become gripped by a strong ongoing negative emotion (fear, despair, hopelessness, etc.).

- Develop an overall sense of despair, powerlessness, helplessness and hopelessness.
- Have others in his social environment that shared similar negative beliefs and expectations.

If all the above criteria were met, Dr. Cannon noted that the person would likely die. Now, you may ask, how does this relate to a serious illness such as cancer?

SUGGESTIBILITY

When a person, overnight, goes from having total faith in his body's ability to be well, to being diagnosed with a serious or terminal condition, the rug is brutally pulled from under him. Chaos prevails. A flood of strong negative emotions arrives. What was of little interest yesterday becomes today's preoccupation or obsession. Conventional theory in psychology suggests that in the presence of extreme negative emotion, a person may lose their normal levels of critical evaluation and become highly susceptible to accepting suggestion. This phenomenon can be used to beneficial effect using hypnosis. (*See* page 34)

NEGATIVE BELIEF AND EXPECTATION

As humans, we are constantly receiving information regarding diseases, their treatment and likely outcomes. This comes from friends, family, neighbours, newspapers, television, internet, etc. We all, therefore, tend to have well-established preconceptions about the outcome of these ailments. We 'know' what is likely to happen. If such a diagnosis arrives, these preconceptions rush to the forefront of the mind. They will almost certainly lead to strong negative beliefs and expectations. The patient receiving the prognosis may well not even hear the 'good' aspects of the diagnosis/prognosis but find himself catapulted inwards to his prior knowledge of the condition and its likely outcome (generally negative).

STRONG NEGATIVE EMOTION

When told of a serious or terminal condition, a patient invariably experiences a range of strong negative emotions. The strongest emotions tend to be fear, closely followed by confusion. This is why you hear people talk about 'blind' fear or 'blind' anger. Rational critical thinking is lost. This means that a patient may well accept an 'apparent' suggestion of doom (which is often not founded in fact).

POWERLESSNESS

Dr Lydia Temoshok identified powerless, helplessness and hopelessness as frequent co-contributors to the onset, development and progression of cancer. These particular emotions are frequently present in patients with serious conditions both at the diagnosis, prognosis and treatment stages but particularly in the weeks and months following treatment.

SOCIAL BELIEFS

Because the public at large have cultural beliefs and expectations about diseases such as cancer, a patient's friends, family and neighbours bring their own preconceptions and expectations to bear, and may begin to treat him as an 'ill' person. Many social beliefs are communicated outside of consciousness through subtle behaviours and responses. Some patients decide to keep their disease status private and there may well be some wisdom in this, as it inhibits those we interact with from potentially influencing the outcome in a negative way.

I recall a patient who was HIV positive, but in robust health, being asked by a medical receptionist, 'Are you still managing the stairs?' Having just returned from a very active skiing trip, she was able to see the irony in this unsubtle message. However, interactions like this tend to re-enforce the patient's own negative beliefs and expectations, thereby creating a closed loop. The same will apply to the preconceptions of the GP and specialists, and their private thoughts about a prognosis are often communicated to the patient indirectly.

PRESTIGE PERSON

In the absence of having personal expert knowledge about any given disease, a patient will tend to defer to the 'expert', accepting what is said as fact, even though it is always only an opinion. The negative beliefs taken on board, following consultation with a doctor or consultant, can take root in the psyche just as surely as the witch doctor's curse, with similar potentially disastrous consequences. To quote a client of ours whose consultant had told him to go and attend to his affairs: 'In one moment it was like being in the Sahara Desert . . . no water for days . . . pressure in the head . . . Where do I go now?'

Doctors are particularly vulnerable when they become patients themselves. We have worked with a number of doctors who, personally, were dealing with cancer in their own bodies. They reported that they would never have believed the devastating effect of a consultant's words on a patient had they not, themselves, been at the receiving end.

It is an accepted fact that in the presence of a strong negative emotion, the unconscious mind is open to accepting suggestion, from others or from self, without the presence of normal critical judgement. This phenomenon will not happen if you have an awareness of that potential, and take appropriate action to correct this in the event that it does happen.

In July 2004, Health Minister, Mr. Michael Martin stated 'Cancer is not only a physical disease. A diagnosis of cancer can be associated with significant psychological morbidity.' This has led him to prioritise the opening of psychooncology units at St. James's and St. Vincent's hospitals in Dublin.

Doctors will admit that many patients tend to die 'on schedule' in or about the time-scale allotted. Given what has been described above in relation to beliefs, verified by Dr. Cannon's research on witch doctors, could it be that we have extraordinarily accurate prognosticians? Or could it be that beliefs and expectations about a prognosis might sometimes play a part in a self-fulfilling prophesy. Think about it!

NO DOCTOR BASHING

A doctor is required by professional ethics to make essential information available to a patient even if this is 'bad' news. However, Hippocrates said, 'First do no harm.' Doctors and consultants do their best to follow this medical maxim. In principle, they try to satisfy themselves that they are doing everything to avoid the 'self-fulfilling voodoo prophesy' scenario previously described. However, this is not always the case.

A challenge of modern medicine is the shortage of time between doctor and patient, time even for full information to be discussed. Equally, there is little time for assisting the patient to come to terms, psychologically, with the diagnosis, and to develop a well-formed strategy for dealing with it. Most doctors have no specific training in this area. As health budgets soar out of control, this time-pressure is increasing, meaning that the psychological and emotional aspects are often neglected. This is not the result of some mal-intent on the part of the doctor but simply due to scarcity of resources.

This aspect cannot reasonably be said to be the exclusive responsibility of the medical staff. It is up to the patient to identify if such unhelpful ideas or beliefs have been accepted into the unconscious mind and, if so, to correct them.

How can you evaluate your diagnosis and prognosis, given the potential time-bomb which may have been activated through inadvertent acceptance of unhelpful beliefs. In an ideal world, to avoid the risk of accepting such potentially dangerous ideas, the patient would be given the following information as a solution:

1. **What is the worst that can happen?**
   'The tests have revealed that you have advanced prostate cancer; at this stage you may have as little as nine months.' (Patient often goes inside and stops hearing at this stage.)
2. **What is the mean or average?**
   'The average survival time for a person of your age and condition with this form of cancer, if treated, is 20–24 months.' (Patient unfortunately often accepts this as *fact*.)
3. **What is the best that can happen?**
   'I have several patients in this city who have had this condition for over fifteen years and they are alive and well.' (Patient rarely hears such positive information if offered).

'Our job as patient and physician is to find where in the spectrum of outcomes we can get you to, to use all possible ways to improve the odds of your getting into that 'winners circle'.'

If the diagnosis/prognosis is communicated in this way, the risk of medical hexing is minimised. Also when consultants record the diagnosis/prognosis on audiotape for a patient, this too eliminates risk of the same. Feel free to ask for it.

DISTANT CONSULTANTS

A majority of doctors entered medicine because they cared about people and wanted to help the human condition. They go through 7 to 10 years of harsh and demanding training learning good science. A doctor told me recently that, apart from the inhuman hours and workload, a doctor in training must learn up to 15,000 unfamiliar words or expressions. When you consider a working vocabulary for a language is perhaps 3,000 words, it gives an idea of the wringer through which doctors are processed in training. After all this, they may go on to specialise, devoting perhaps a further 7 to 12 years to further training to bring their particular skills to the highest level.

However, they then have to contend with the harsh reality that what they know is not always enough, and patients will die or deteriorate anyway. For someone who has spent more than 20 years in training, who really cares about the welfare of patients, this can be the ultimate insult to a doctor's skills and knowledge. The patient deteriorates or dies in spite of their best efforts.

Patients might consider having a degree of compassion for the sense of helplessness a doctor has in such a situation. Is it any wonder that doctors have higher levels of alcoholism, drug addiction, relationship problems and live shorter lives than do the general population. Is it any wonder that, to protect themselves from the pain and hurt of losing a patient, consultants often retreat behind a mask of apparent coldness and 'professional' detachment?

Whilst looking to understand and have compassion for the medical profession, you also have to consider yourself. If you have been given a diagnosis of serious illness and you want to get into that 'winners circle', then you must check as to whether unhelpful beliefs have inadvertently been introduced into your psyche and which now may be a 'dripping battery acid' creating that self-fulfilling prophesy. Working with a skilled therapist can help identify and re-balance such potential negative and toxic beliefs.

Dr. Larry LeShan has been carrying out pioneering clinical research work in behavioural medicine for almost half a century. He states:

> Nobody has the right to attack or weaken a persons defences (hopes) unless those conditions are seriously interfering with their ability to deal with the illness. Since 1955, literally dozens of studies have shown conclusively that emotional life history often does play an important part in determining an individual's resistance to getting cancer and in how the cancer develops after it appears. Since I learned to use a psychotherapeutic approach, over a 20-year period, approximately half of my 'hopeless' patients have gone into long-term remission and are still alive.

Because of their vulnerable state (in our experience), patients often misinterpret the sometimes-distant attitude of consultants and specialists as either rejection or negativity regarding the outcomes of their disease. It is important for the patient to review such a response. In your consultant or specialist, you have a potent source of expertise and access to many years of experience. However, a negative or remote attitude has the possibility of provoking an unhelpful (and consequential hormonal) response in you. If this is so, it is your responsibility, as the patient, to notice and correct this.

~ SUMMARY ~

A doctor's negative beliefs and expectations can kill you.
A doctor's positive beliefs and expectations can heal you.

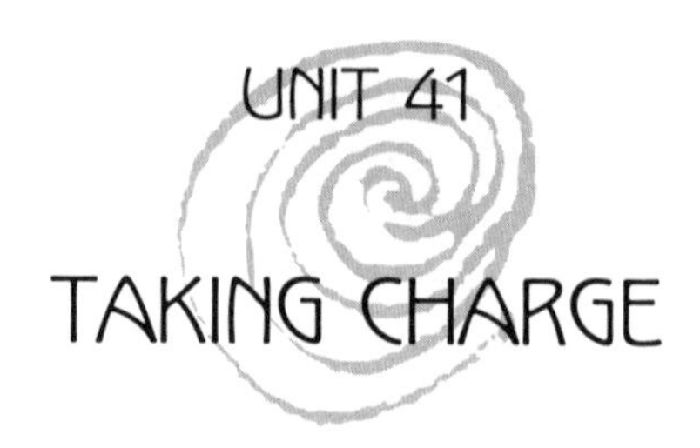

UNIT 41

TAKING CHARGE

To move away from any sense of powerlessness and given that, if things go wrong, it is you who will pay the price, why not give a thought to taking charge? When did you last call a case conference? Who is in charge of your case? Are you given access to the results of tests, access to medical records? A technician may not give you factual information but fob you off with, 'Ask your doctor.' Any theft of your independence and personal power, removal of clothes, access to phones, etc., can foster a sense of helplessness and negatively affect your immune system. The job of your medical team is to give encouragement and inspiration. Do you have access to trained psychotherapists and counsellors? Have you access to a Behavioural Medicine programme?

PERSONAL RESPONSIBILITY

Psychological interventions are often not used in the treatment of cancer in case the patient might be made to feel guilty about being responsible for the development of the disease. However psychologist Fred Gallo, Ph.D. suggests, 'You cannot change a problem in your life unless you are willing to accept that to some degree you were involved in creating it.' If you live in a simplistic world of single causes and effects, this comment might be valid. The reality is, diseases such as cancer and heart disease have been clearly shown to be complex and multi-causal. In most instances patients play some part in its origins, but this does not make them solely responsible.

The obligation of medicine is to provide the patients with the support and skills to follow a healthy lifestyle. It is unacceptable that doctors 'collude' with patients in not insisting that this lifestyle change be part of their medical programme.

Drugs have enabled us to turn off much of the feedback (e.g. pain, anxiety etc.) from the body that tells us that we need to change the way we are living. Because of this, the concept of health is becoming more detached from the actuality of our lifestyles. The reality is that healthcare is a privilege, and privileges carry responsibility. This responsibility rests with the partnership of patient and doctor, and both have an equal part to play in seeking recovery.

No patient we have ever come across is wholly responsible for his condition. However, as stated, most will have made some contribution to it. This is not a reason for guilt but rather a cause for celebration because if they have participated in their illness they now have the power to participate in its resolution. Unfortunately, therapists and doctors concerned about eliciting a guilt response, have been reluctant to confront their patients with this opportunity to take positive life-changing action.

With regard to personal responsibility, the paradox remains that 'saints' have died of cancer and other conditions, while 'sinners' go on to live long lives – there is a mystery here. Sometimes disease is just a part of the human experience. However, to succumb to a condition, leaving many evidence-based stones unturned, is folly. Our job as humans and authors is to create an optimum physical, emotional and spiritual environment, combined with the wonders of modern medicine, and then see what Mother Nature has to offer.

The World Health Organisation says, 'People not only have the right to participate individually and collectively in the planning and implementation of health care programmes, but also have a duty to do so.'

LOCUS OF CONTROL

Numerous studies have shown that chronic feelings of helplessness and hopelessness lower immune response. The old medical model sought to remove a patient's perception of sense of control. An example would be the removal of clothes, limiting of visitors, etc. The opposite of this, which psychologists call 'positive (or internal) locus of control' has been demonstrated to improve immune response. The new thinking acknowledges this, but to date offers no specific training in how to capitalise on the positive effect of a 'sense of personal control'. Part of a Behavioural Medicine coaching programme sets out specifically to encourage this locus of control.

MEMBERSHIP OF A 'NEW CLUB' AND PEER SUPPORT

Most people live their daily lives in a sense of immortality. In the *Bhagavad-Gita*, Krishna is reputed to have asked Arjuna, 'What is the most amazing thing about people?' The response: 'That people can live their daily lives surrounded by death and yet be able to pretend that it will not happen to them.'

If you have been diagnosed with a serious illness then, like it or not, you have become a member of a new club whose members, at least for the moment, can no longer sustain the illusion of immortality. When you personally face death or severe incapacity, this makes you interact with other people differently; your priorities and life goals may change overnight.

This is important for the special people in your life in that they may find it difficult to understand your altered thinking and feelings, your new way of experiencing life. Unless people themselves have been put in a position of confronting their own mortality, it is unlikely they will be able to truly empathise or understand what is going on in your world. These special people in your life are important to you, however, because you love them and they love you. They are also a vital element in your support system when confronting the illness, so it is critical to offer them some understanding on this aspect so that when you recover the relationships remain intact and you can move forward to even stronger ones.

I have found that this aspect of an illness reveals the particular value of working in a support group. You can find space to discuss such challenging issues in a supportive environment with people who will understand much of what you are dealing with. Off-loading frustrations in a 'safe' place means that you can go back to your loved-ones, free of resentment and feeling much more clear-headed and positive about what you expect of them and what you are able to give in return.

You must also demand that a support system be put in place for close family members to get help, not only for themselves, but to help them in their role of supporting you.

~ SUMMARY ~

If you don't take control of your own recovery, then who will?

KEY NOTES

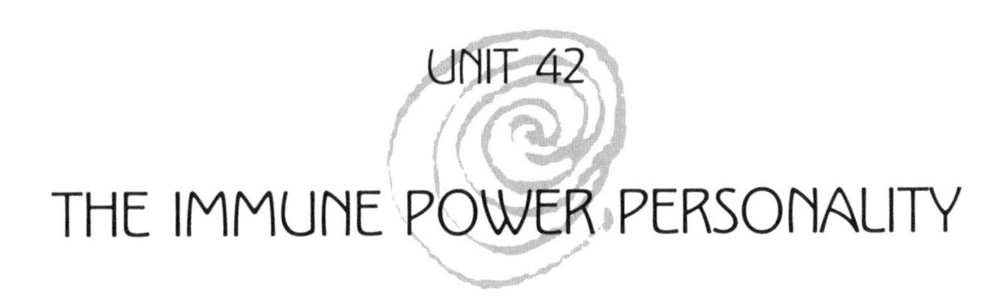

UNIT 42

THE IMMUNE POWER PERSONALITY

'Everybody has a basic nature and we have an acquired nature and it's hard sometimes to tell the difference.'
CHARLES TART, PH.D.

In 1997, while walking in Glendalough with a colleague, Deirdre Davis Brigham, we were introduced to the concept of an Immune Power Personality. Current research suggests there are some people who possess specific personality traits (habitual ways of being) that are helpful in stimulating immune function which makes them 'miracle-prone', and others have traits that are unhelpful (please note we did not say 'good' or 'bad') which make them 'disease-prone'. The research suggests that positive traits are potentialities in all of us, and can be awakened through awareness, short-term therapy and practice.

In case readers start feeling guilty about their personality traits, we can assure you that nobody in their right mind sets out to create a disease or illness for himself. We don't receive an owner's manual when we're born and, as children, we don't have the gift of foresight. It's not surprising that we often develop 'unhelpful' personality traits.

As infants, we begin to adapt to the world around us. We notice that crying brings food and comfort, and later on we use that behaviour to get parental attention. At the toddler stage we discover which behaviours bring us smiles and rewards and which bring punishment. Little girls are encouraged to be kind, caring, meek and obedient; little boys are rewarded for being brave, tough and competitive and for 'not crying'.

Strange as it may seem, these personality traits, developed to help us survive the trials of childhood, are often those that, if taken to the extreme in adult life, may predispose us to serious illness. Acknowledging possession of such traits can now enable us to review and change them. If they are causing a problem in our lives, we can get professional help from counselling or psychotherapy, or from a good life-skills training programme.

Barbara Levine writes, 'Predictive studies following students over 30 years showed personality-predicted vulnerability to cancer, heart disease and blood pressure.'

The following distinct but overlapping concepts are the result of extensive scientific studies. With the exceptions of Alan Luks (whose work has been validated elsewhere), all are psychologists or psychiatrists of note who have conducted original studies published in leading scientific journals. These concepts are:

Attend, Connect and Express
People who actually notice or attend to their own mind-body signals of discomfort, pain, fatigue, distress, sadness, anger, and pleasure, cope better and have better immune profiles and a healthier cardiovascular system, according to Psychologist, Gary Schwartz, Ph.D., of University of Arizona.

Capacity to Confide
James Pennebaker, Ph.D., demonstrated that individuals who confide their secrets, traumas and feelings to themselves and others have a livelier immune response, healthier psychological profiles, faster recovery from illness, and far fewer incidences of illness.

Hardiness, Commitment, Control and Challenge
Susanne Ouellette, Ph.D., a psychologist at the City University of New York, originated the concept of 'personality hardiness'. This quality which causes people to experience fewer chronic illnesses and symptoms and have stronger immune systems comes from the '3 Cs': 1. A sense of **Control** over one's quality of life, health and social conditions; 2. A strong **Commitment** to one's work, creative activities, or relationships; and 3. A view of stress or disease as a **Challenge** rather than a threat. Threat and Challenge produce different responses in the body.

Assertiveness
George F. Solomon, M.D., an early pioneer in the field of Psychoneuroimmunology (PNI), conducted some of the earliest studies on personality and immunity. He showed that people who assert their needs and feelings have stronger and more balanced

immune responses. They more readily resist and overcome a range of diseases associated with dysfunctional immunity – from rheumatoid arthritis to AIDS.

Affiliative Trust

David McLelland, Ph.D., a world renowned psychologist of Boston University, has discovered that individuals who are strongly motivated to form relationships with others based on unconditional love and trust, rather than frustrated power, have more vigorous immune systems and reduced incidence of illness.

Healthy Helping and Altruism

Health Investigator, Alan Luks, conducted a large survey showing that people committed to helping others, displaying the personality trait of altruism, suffer far fewer illnesses and recover faster.

Self-Complexity

Patricia Linville, a psychologist at Duke University, has demonstrated that people who explore many facets of their personality, called 'self-aspects' (or explore what it means to be human), can better withstand stressful life circumstances. These people are less prone to stress, depression, physical symptoms and infections in the wake of such stressful life events.

~ SUMMARY ~

Winners in wellness-recovery have distinctive personality traits.

KEY NOTES

UNIT 43

CHARACTERISTICS OF THE MIRACLE PRONE

The following are common characteristics identified in over 2,500 so-called 'miracle' cases of spontaneous remission from illness reported in medical journals.

- To have an **open mind**, to want to be cured, but not to approach fighting back with this as the single-minded purpose of their journey.
- To be in a state of psychological void, with an openness to paradox, mystery and the fullness of life.
- To have made, or be making, a shift from dependency to autonomy. Noticing a subtle change in belief system from feeling 'out of control' to feeling that the process of healing comes from within rather than without.
- To have made spiritual changes involving connection of mind, body and spirit.
- To have a confidence and awareness beyond the rational, logical, simplistic knowledge of everyday life.
- To possess a yearning for much more from life than mere coping, survival, success and security. To transcend the here and now, actively searching for the meaning of life.
- To have a tendency to be a psychic gambler, a willingness to take risks for the fulfilment of dreams, and a predilection to think in a freewheeling style that reflects the uncertainty of life. To be flexible and adaptable, emotionally biphasic and paradoxical, with strong mood fluctuations. That is: to express feelings and to be as passionate about grief as about joy. Being expressive about the disease is a key aspect.
- 'They're not one way or the other. They are both one way and the other – logical and intuitive; confident and self-critical; co-operative and rebellious; spiritual and irreverent; consistent and unpredictable; hopeful and despairing'.
- They are complex and paradoxical. They acknowledge the contradictory parts of themselves, are comfortable with who they are and find their own songs to sing rather than imitating the songs of others who have been healed. (There's no point in using the neighbour's key to open your door! It is a key but it is unique!)

- The biggest barrier to developing a 'survivor' personality comes from having been raised a 'nice' person. (One patient said, 'How do I break out?')

(Grateful thanks to O'Regan, Hirshberg, Siebert and Pearsall)

~ SUMMARY ~

Extraordinary survivors have personality traits which are learnable.

KEY NOTES

'The programme enabled me to think about my illness at a deeper level, in that it helped me to understand the incredible emotions I had to deal with on hearing I had cancer, ... I was able to take back the power that lies deep within me and recognise I could play a big part in healing myself – which I did!' *P. McM., Dublin*

UNIT 44

STRESS AND CRITICAL MASS

We have all heard of the concept of the last straw that breaks the camel's back. We know the body has a miraculous capacity to tolerate the inevitable stresses of life. However, there comes a time when you may have taken on 'one straw too many', you have no reserves left and you just can't cope with it.

Which is the 'straw' which when removed, stops the camel's back from being threatened with breaking? The answer is that it doesn't really matter. Removing just about any straw (or stressor) will do the job.

In general, someone becomes overweight by eating too much or not exercising enough. How then can a person loose weight? The choices are to exercise more or eat less or both. By doing this, they open up the capacity to be able to take in more food yet not put on weight. Stress is no different. If we experience excessive stress or a lot of little stresses, unless we have reserve capacity, then the resources of the body are at risk of overwhelm and, as Hans Selye said, 'exhaustion and death follow'.

The choices are to create some additional reserves, given that diagnosis and treatments will inevitably bring more stress challenges. This 'reserve' capacity can be created effectively through many of the Behavioural Medicine techniques described here.

~ SUMMARY ~

Sometimes it is the last tiny change you make in something that makes the crucial difference.

UNIT 45

FOUR STAGES OF LEARNING & KNOWLEDGE VERSUS SKILL

Responding to a serious illness often involves learning new skills. Unfortunately, this tends to be at the very time when perhaps you are feeling worried, frightened, angry or impatient. We find, therefore, that health-challenged patients have difficulty in engaging with enthusiasm in acquiring new skills. If you find yourself 'stuck', going backwards, or unable to move forward, then beating yourself up or berating your performance will only make things worse.

STAGES OF LEARNING A SKILL ARE

Stage 1: **Unconscious Incompetence:** This is when you are unable to perform some task or activity and you can't think of any reason why you would want to.

Stage 2: **Conscious Incompetence:** This is when you now become aware of the need to be able to perform some new task or activity yet, when you try it, your performance is poor or disappointing. Many people use this phase to focus on their supposed lack of ability, and sometimes even try to skip this phase altogether. Few give themselves permission to recognise this as an essential stage in achieving excellence in anything.

Stage 3: **Conscious Competence:** This is when a person, through coaching and practice, is able to perform the required task or activity reasonably well. However they have to retain a lot of conscious and 'self-conscious' involvement in the activity, thereby performing below their optimum capability.

Stage 4: **Unconscious Competence:** This is when, having practiced, learned, and corrected, someone is able to relinquish conscious involvement in a process and just get on with doing the job excellently.

Regardless of the context, it is useful to allow yourself to return to the Conscious Incompetence stage, purposefully, allowing yourself to flounder about and re-learn what you need to learn, so that you can motivate yourself to do what your body/mind needs to recover. We have heard of world-class sportsmen doing just that when they go off form.

~ SUMMARY ~

Learning new life skills is a process and not an event.

KEY NOTES

'My participation in the Behavioural Medicine programme gave me a sense of self-esteem which I found very beneficial. I also found that participation in the group situation was very helpful and encouraging.' *R.B., Co. Dublin*

UNIT 46

THE DOCTOR-PATIENT RELATIONSHIP

Studies show that a majority of people (80-90%) with diseases, who engage in complementary or alternative approaches, do not tell their doctor what they are doing. This seems to be because they are afraid of having their hopes and ideas belittled or scoffed at. A frequent response from doctors tends to be 'Well... (long pause) hmmm . . . it probably won't do you any harm.' (Please note the unspoken presupposition: 'It probably won't do you any good either!')

In so far as is possible, work only with a doctor who is willing to respect your right to participate actively in your own recovery. If your doctor or consultant does not respect this right, perhaps it is time to review the composition of your medical team.

To be successful in a 'fight back' programme, it is essential that you discuss with your doctors all complementary approaches you are using, even if they don't believe in them. You are free to request, 'If in your professional opinion, a specific complementary treatment doesn't represent a risk to me, and is unlikely to interfere in my medical treatment, then please keep your counsel and allow me to make my own judgement' . . . and that includes the very expressive 'shrug of the shoulders'.

Your GP's support is important; he is nearby when consultants are not. If you don't have complete confidence in him, or you don't find him supportive – then find a new GP.

A doctor is a potent source of accurate information and treatment. However, he is also your 'employee'. You pay his wages (or the Government does) to provide you with specialist knowledge and skills. However, as a fellow human being, he is also expected to provide you with caring, respect, fairness and understanding. We are shocked at how patients still describe how often these qualities are lacking. We recall one patient who met her surgeon (who had previously removed her stomach due to cancer) in the lobby of a large Dublin hospital. When he asked, 'How are you?' she said, 'I've had a recurrence, this time in the liver.' His reply was: 'This is hardly the place to discuss this,' and he walked away, leaving her shattered. Fortunately these thoughtless people are in a minority – but they still have the opportunity to do serious psychological damage.

THE PATIENT ASKS . . .

Doctors and consultants . . . do please:

- Be careful of what you say. 'We didn't find too many big tumours this time.' can be heard as, '...We found a million small ones!'
- If you are feeling negative, please keep it to yourself. It does not serve me unless it is balanced by an authentic belief in my potential. Remember, I hang on your on your every word!
- Allow me to participate in the management of my illness. I am the one who will live with the consequences.
- Do not think that you have all the answers.
- Give me proof (including studies and reports) that the interventions you recommend will cure my condition, or at least extend my life expectancy and quality of life. Remember, I have a right to receive this information.
- Allow me space to talk about complementary treatments I may wish to explore. If, in your professional opinion, such treatments don't represent a risk to me or will not interfere in my medical treatment, then allow me to make my own judgement. Don't undermine my faith in their validity
- You have the skills and training to diagnose and to make a prognosis. I have the right to know what the worst-case and best-case scenarios are. We, together, will determine to what point on the spectrum of possibility I might reach. (Please remember, nobody has the right to sentence me!)

THE DOCTOR ASKS . . .

The Doctor asks . . . Patients do please:

- Prepare your questions in advance of a consultation (so you leave with the important ones answered). It's OK to give them to me written down or to post them in advance. Obligations to other patients will probably limit the time I can give you to answer questions so prioritise your questions.
- Beware of interpreting a casual 'throw-away' comment from me. If you're not sure, ask!
- Do not pretend you understand if you don't. Demand clarification!
- Make sure you understand the purpose of your medication, the dosage and the frequency.
- Report all unusual symptoms or possible side-effects. If necessary, write them down in advance.

- Your friends, family, or neighbours are neither physicians nor diagnosticians. Please do not rely on them for professional information or advice. If there is confusion, ask me for clarification. Avoid taking notice of 'old-wives-tales', or taking advice meant for others.
- Do not mix medications. Do not take natural herbs, vitamins, minerals or over-the-counter drugs without advising me. Even if I don't approve, I need to know! (Mega-doses of vitamins and minerals can sometimes interfere with medications or treatments such as chemotherapy, so check!) Ask me for current research references (rather than my personal opinion).
- Expect caring, respect, fairness and understanding.
- Communicate what you want and what your expectations are, and ask for as much information as you need.
- Follow my prescriptions and recommendations. You are free to decline, but do, please, let me know!
- Feel free to ask for a second opinion. I am not offended by such thoroughness and would be happy to help you find one.
- Feel free to ask (and if necessary, insist on knowing) 'What's the longest time anyone has survived with this illness with quality of life?' or 'What's the shortest time anyone has taken to heal from this?' If I don't know, insist that I find out!
- Feel free to question tests, medications, their necessity and frequency. The 'body' in question is yours – you have the right to decide what happens to it!
- Remember, when you have an appointment to see me, check with my staff at least ten days before your visit, to see if medical tests are required. We can then make the most of the consultation. This will save dragging you back unnecessarily. I am human, so do your part.

~ SUMMARY ~

You can dramatically enhance the benefits you get from your medical team through effective communication.

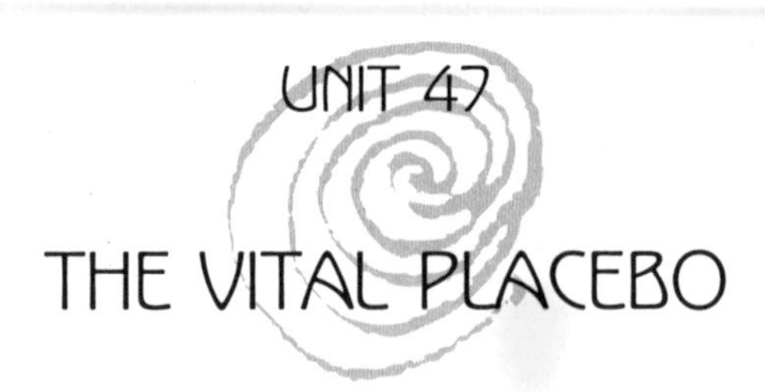

UNIT 47

THE VITAL PLACEBO

Doctors are trained in careful science. The scientific method demands the statement of a problem, the formation of a hypothesis or theory, observation and experimentation, interpretation of data and the drawing of conclusions. The evolution of this scientific method was to protect the patient from the exploitation of charlatans and 'snake-oil' salesmen (who it appeared may have, unwittingly, harnessed the mysteries of the placebo effect). However, the psychological and spiritual aspects of man don't easily lend themselves to objective measurement.

When people are listening to emotionally-charged information about themselves, research suggests that they hear 100% of the first chunk, 70% of the second and perhaps 40% of the third. The potential good news is often late in the communication – and often goes unheard.

It is only in the last twenty to thirty years that the human immune system has begun to yield up some of its secrets. It has been shown conclusively that the brain, the mind, and the body are part of the same system and that what affects one part will affect all in a closed cybernetic (feed-back) loop. When the body is negatively affected, the mind responds. When the mind is negatively affected, the body responds.

The 'placebo' is a human phenomenon observed over centuries and, until the evolution of the scientific testing for drugs, was believed to have been responsible for much of the effectiveness of many old 'medicines'. One Internet search engine, recently, had almost three million references to 'placebo'! The phenomenon is such that if a person takes an inert or chemically neutral substance, yet has strong belief and expectation of a positive result, their body will produce that result in a significant number of cases – typically at 50%. For instance, if an asthmatic is given something harmless such as rosewater as an inhalant, but believes it to be a new potent broncho-dilator, it will often halt an asthma attack. However, if something is known to be a placebo, it will not work.

The statistics for the effectiveness of placebo, as described above, will produce a significant clinical effect in at least 35–50% of people. Professor Herbert Benson of Harvard University and Dr. Alan Roberts of Scripps Clinic in California suggest this now can be as high as 70%.

In the October 2002 edition of '*Health Which?*', the UK Consumers' Association published results of a recent report by a team from the University of Connecticut (led by Professor Irving Kirsch) suggesting that only 18% of the response to the six most widely prescribed antidepressant drugs is due to the medication itself; a massive 82% of the response is duplicated in patients taking a placebo.

The word placebo means: 'I shall please' in Latin. Its mechanisms remain a mystery, but its power is none the less potent. It appears that the human body possesses an ability to transform positive belief and expectation into potent hormones and chemicals as part of its natural self-healing mechanism.

There have been cases where patients with cancer were inadvertently told, due to a mix-up in X-rays, that their cancer was gone. When the mix-up was subsequently discovered and the people were checked, the cancer had disappeared completely! A famous case from the annals of medical history was a certain Mr. Wright, who was suffering with late-stage terminal cancer. He had been assessed as having only weeks to live. He talked his way onto a test panel for a new experimental anti-cancer drug called Krebiozen. Within a week of receiving the drug, his cancer specialist described Mr. Wright's tumours as shrinking 'like snowballs in a hot oven' and he went into complete remission. Some months later, doubts were expressed in the media about the efficacy of Krebiozen. Mr Wright's tumours returned almost immediately. His oncologist, who had been amazed at the original disappearance, now engaged in a deception (which, ethically, would not be acceptable today). He informed Mr. Wright that the original batch of Krebiozen had been 'defective' in some way, and would Mr. Wright like to receive the new 'super enhanced' Krebiozen? Mr Wright enthusiastically agreed.

There was no 'super' Krebiozen and what the doctor actually injected was sterile water. Mr. Wright's tumours again disappeared and he returned to his normal life. Three months later, an announcement was made in the medical media that Krebiozen was judged to be worthless. Mr Wright learned of this, his tumours returned almost immediately, and he died shortly afterwards.

It is now a requirement that all new drugs be subjected to rigorous double-blind clinical trials. After preliminary studies on animals, a double blind controlled study is carried out. Volunteer patients are asked to participate in the trial. Some will be given the real drug being tested, some will be given the next best-known alternative drug and some will receive a placebo (an inert substance disguised as the real drug). None of the medical or research personnel will know which is the real drug and which is the placebo. This type of study was introduced because it was shown that patients would pick up the tiniest gesture or eye movement that would tell if the doctor was hopeful or pessimistic, and this would then skew the research data.

If these micro signs are so important in research, how significant are the beliefs and expectations of your medical personnel in your recovery?

Researcher, Dr. Ernest Rossi reported research showing that over 30% of medical prescriptions in England were, in effect, placebo in that the drugs could not have any specific physiological effect on the conditions for which they were prescribed. Research in the United States suggested a similar figure. Additionally, research suggests that, 50% of the time, sub-clinical dosages of medicines often produce the full clinical effect, again, it would appear, based on activation of the placebo mechanism. The Office of Technology Assessments in the US reported that only 17–20% of conventional medical practices are based on scientifically validated evidence, so there remains, perhaps, a vast area of unnoticed potential placebo activity here.

Although, as stated, placebo is used in drug trials, science tends to dismiss the effect because we do not understand the mechanisms involved. It is a mystery. If the placebo effect has long since been shown to work, why should we not be willing to live with paradox, maintain good standards of science and concurrently remain open to mystery?

If this miraculous capability in the human body-mind has been demonstrated to exist, as evidenced by its requirement in medical drug trials, why then is it not exploited in the modern treatment of disease? Perhaps on the emergence of science-based medications, doctors wanted to distance themselves from the murky past of sugar pills and potions. They wanted everything to be based on 'good science'. However in the process of separating the body from the mind and the spirit, we believe that doctors may have mislaid one of the body's greatest wonders, the capacity to use its own chemistry laboratory and chemist shop to produce needed chemicals or drugs.

Doctors are sceptical about any treatment that appears to rely on the expectations of therapist and patient for its effectiveness. The placebo effect is also criticised as being unreliable, as it seemed to affect only 35–50% of patients. Perhaps the placebo effect is always available if we can provide the appropriate environment within which it can be activated! One doctor quipped to us, 'Placebo is what happens when other doctors succeed with your failures!'

Nobody is suggesting that patients should intentionally be given false drugs or sham treatments. However this is very different from the patients finding their own objects of belief, hope and expectation and, provided they are not contraindicated, they may then become a trigger for the body's own self-healing mechanism.

Because most medical interventions are inherently dangerous, they must be treated as 'guilty until proven innocent'. Because most alternative or complementary approaches are inherently benign, and have a good possibility of triggering the 40–70% placebo effect, perhaps they might now be treated as 'innocent until proven guilty!'

Unfortunately, we hear from patients that they often do not tell doctors about their secret 'potions' (placebo triggers). They describe proposing something to their doctor and get the response, 'It won't do you any harm – try it if you like, but I think you're wasting your time.' Sometimes these 'potions' have a clinical effect, and sometimes they are activating placebo effect. The doctor's words, although well intentioned, are frequently offered in a scornful tone and an attitude of dismissal. Since we have known for centuries that the placebo effect exists, that it affects up to perhaps 70% of people, it may now border on the unethical to dismiss such treatments without objective justification.

The negative side of concealing these complementary approaches from your doctor is that some of them can actually interfere with the effectiveness of the mainstream medical approach, such as boosting immune function concurrent with receiving chemotherapy, (which is designed in fact to deplete it). Such treatments may be an absolute requirement prior to and after chemotherapy, but not during. Unless there is a trusting and open relationship between doctor and patient, they may inadvertently work against each other.

Dr. Larry Dossey, M.D., comments, 'If the placebo effect is required as part of the gold standard in double-blind testing of drugs, why is it that no effort has been given to looking at ways to engage, encourage, enhance this effect or potentate it or study it, given that for 35%-70% of patients, circumstances can trigger the self-healing mechanism?'

We have read studies on alternative treatments that were proving quite effective for a proportion of patients, and were not harmful. However, as soon as they were subjected to double-blind controlled studies and shown to be no more effective than placebo, they then became useless (loss of belief and expectation), and an opportunity had been lost. How sad!

Any double-blind study that excludes the psychological perspective is deficient! It only evidences what works for people with certain pre-existing psychological configurations. Lots of patients often project healing capability onto all sorts of spurious stuff and bingo! They enable their body, via the mind, to produce a positive effect.

Professor Benson suggests that the elements necessary for triggering a placebo response are:

- Belief and expectation on the part of the patient.
- Belief and expectancy on the part of the therapist/physician.

Therefore, your job as a patient is to seek to establish both. The placebo effect is almost always detected retrospectively. If a person knows it is a placebo, it will not work. However we can create environments in which it can occur spontaneously and naturally.

THE NOCEBO EFFECT

'Nocebo', as described by Professor Herbert Benson of Harvard, operates to the same principles as placebo. However in this instance, it operates in the opposite direction. The body produces a destructive reaction in response to imagination, belief and expectation, and herein lies significant risk for the patient.

Clinical trials have shown that approximately 35% of patients will experience hair loss if they receive an injection of a harmless saline solution – provided they believe it is potent chemotherapy and that they expect such hair loss! Equally, asthmatics sensitive to something like a rose will often have a real attack when in the presence of such a flower, even though afterwards it is shown to be just a cleverly crafted silk imitation.

Another amazing phenomenon has emerged in research. When patients are given a 'proven' medication, but it is suggested to them, directly or indirectly, that it is 'only a placebo', in 30–40% of cases, the patient will experience no clinical benefit – in other words, the body manages to negate the clinical effect! If our asthmatic is given some powerful drug, but believes it to be useless, it will often have no beneficial effect. Here we have vivid demonstrations of the power of negative belief and expectation. The Coroner of Baltimore once commented on the number of people who had intentionally or inadvertently taken poison, but having taken quantities so small as to be harmless, yet they died, thanks to the power of belief and expectation!

A recent book entitled *Snake Oil*, by John Diamond, places great emphasis on the fact that many complementary therapies are based solely on belief and expectation. He himself admitted to having neither, and hence found that they did not work for him. He paid the price for having an exceptionally sceptical attitude – the placebo effect was not available to him. Doubtless, many therapies have successfully found the mechanism for triggering the placebo healing response in others whose minds provided a more fertile environment!

Elsewhere you will read about the potential risk that may come with diagnosis and prognosis, and the beliefs and expectations emerging at that time. We believe if a physician intentionally or inadvertently cuts away belief and expectation or hope, he may possibly have cut away 30–40% of that person's potential for recovery!

Anyone who produces cures or excellent results, but cannot explain the mechanism, is likely to be condemned. Those cured tend to be ignored; those curing will be attacked. This includes the placebo effect.

In summary, for you the patient, belief and expectation can trigger either a powerful healing response or an injurious one. If you identify therapies that you believe may help, do discuss them with your doctors to check their safety. However, feel free to demand that scorn and scepticism is not what you need if they are deemed safe. Hypnosis and cognitive psychological interventions can enable the harnessing of this in-built ability in humans in about 50% of cases. Dr. Lawrence LeShan, Ph.D., an early pioneer in psycho-behavioural medicine, is on record as stating that over 50% of his patients were alive and well 20 years after receiving a diagnosis of a terminal condition and after engaging in psychotherapy.

As others before us have said: doctors might now begin to heed the potential of 'placebo'. If there is an open honest relationship, then the doctor is the best person with whom to discuss and evaluate other treatments. Unless a doctor knows of some contraindication or risk to the patient, why not encourage the exploration of other treatments with their potential to trigger this potent and proven self-healing mechanism? Sadly I remember one patient with motor neuron disease who asked, 'Would hyberbaric oxygen be useful?' Although this was not contraindicated, she was told, 'Don't waste your money.' Could this have been a placebo opportunity wasted?

FALSE HOPE AND FALSE DESPAIR

Doctors frequently fear being accused of giving a patient false hope. However, as stated elesewhere, Norman Cousins, author of *Anatomy of an Illness* commented, 'There is no such thing as false hope. Hope is a desire for a positive outcome. Despair is the realisation that things may not work out. There is no disease that has killed 100% of the people diagnosed with it!' Accept the diagnosis. Decline the prognosis. Dr. Bernie Siegal commented: 'There is no such thing as false hope, there is only false despair'. All too often, patients are left feeling helpless and hopeless. With so many evidence-based areas for potential exploration, it is arrogant for anybody to suggest that there is nothing more the patient can do.

~ SUMMARY ~

The placebo is a powerful element in your self-healing mechanism.
It can be harnessed.

UNIT 48

PRESUPPOSITIONS AND GENERALISED BELIEFS

Presuppositions are a bit like beliefs. They are not necessarily true. They are simply habitual convenient ways you have evolved of looking at or interacting with the world.

The following are not necessarily true but you might review them. Some are from the world of Neuro-Linguistic Programming (NLP); Others were suggested by former patients. You might consider whether, if you were to adopt some of them, might they impact positively on the progression, regression or cure of your illness?

- Beliefs are only beliefs and not facts. All beliefs can be challenged.
- People have all the ability they need to succeed; there are no unresourceful people, only unresourceful states of mind! If even one person can do something – heal himself or experience remission – then, potentially, you can do it too!
- You, and only you, are in charge of your mind and therefore the results. Professionals may predict your future but only the partnership of patient and doctor can determine it.
- If you always do what you've always done, you'll always get what you always got! If you want something different, then you have to do something different. Survivors almost always radically change many aspects of their lives.
- There is no such thing as 'failure'. Failure can be interpreted as feedback – it offers a unique opportunity to learn something you might otherwise have missed. In other words, keep going.
- Success is the result of good judgement. Good judgement is the result of experience. Experience is often the result of bad judgement.
- You cannot afford the luxury of unaddressed depression.
- Whatever you have done in life, you made the best decisions with the resources, knowledge, and skills you had at the time.
- Ongoing self-blame or self-criticism is useless. Whatever unhelpful behaviours or reactions you once had, learn from them – then let them go.

- The body knows how to heal itself – give it the opportunity.
- The immune system can acquire immunity to any bug if time is made available for the cycle to complete!
- Good news and bad news may both be threatening. (If your prognosis is changed for the better, you may slip back into an unhealthy lifestyle.)
- The mind needs rest AND activity (challenge) for optimum health.
- The body itself can create any drug or hormone it needs.
- Every disease is as unique as the person who has it. Everyone has a self-healing mechanism (SHM) that can be stimulated or suppressed.
- All diseases have survivors and miracles.
- Most diseases originate from a combination of physical, psychological, intellectual, behavioural, environmental, and spiritual factors. Most solutions will likely be the same.
- All unhelpful behaviours, reactions and responses can be changed, but frequently need nudging – and require time.
- 'Experts can predict, but they can never *know* the future.' *(Albert Einstein)*
- Consultant may prognose, but circumstances, action and chance decide.
- You have to build up and maintain reserves of stamina to withstand the inevitable shocks of treatment. This takes time.
- Mind Body and Spirit are part of the same reciprocating system.
- The immune system has the ability to learn (*Robert Ader*).
- The immune system eavesdrops on your internal dialogue.
- No disease kills 100% of people diagnosed with it.
- Not all people exposed to a given condition will contract it.
- Negative information cannot be unheard – but can be re-scripted.
- Disease is a challenge and not a sentence.
- All negative emotions/symptoms are useful feedback to prompt action or awareness.
- We are responsible for our own emotional responses. We just need to develop the skills to manage them.
- When energy is down we need a source of inspiration.
- All personality or coping traits can be changed.
- Energy flows where attention goes. This can be useful or unhelpful – depending on your focus.
- Current belief/behaviour is your best choice for now, but may not be the most useful for the future.
- Underlying all behaviour there is a positive intention. All our internal parts have a positive intent (although this is not always apparent).

- A Behavioural Medicine programme offers a menu of useful proven options; it does not dictate!
- Facts are often ignored if they don't fit with current wisdom.
- The person or system with the most flexibility wins.
- The past tries to dictate the future. Our job is to choose.

You can design your own new beliefs or adopt some of the above although they may not necessarily be 'true'. You can condition them into your psyche by repetition and visualisation. Select the ones that you believe will be useful for you and put them on 3 x 5" cards and carry them about with you – using them regularly as affirmations.

~ SUMMARY ~

Presuppositions are habituated ways of looking at the world.
If they are not helpful, you are free to write a new script.

KEY NOTES

'A maturing and human experience.' J. F. C., Dublin

UNIT 49

WELLNESS AND ITS RISKS

When clients begin to engage in healthier eating, yoga, meditation and other similar approaches, they will often begin to feel better and have more energy, both physically and mentally. In research, we have found this to be a high-risk period. These patients may prematurely begin to take on more, to place more stresses upon themselves. They may stop doing what is making them well. Through this, they may unwittingly squander any gains and put themselves back at square one. There is also a temptation to go into a state of denial about the illness, to act as though it is gone. When you begin to notice this feeling of 'well-ness' returning, as many participants in Behavioural Medicine do, remember this is 'high risk', an alarm bell for caution, a time to engage even more forcefully with your recovery programme!

Once you have had cancer, you will likely always be a person with cancer potential. We have seen patients who have produced spectacular results experience recurrence when they abandon the formula, recipe or wisdom that contributed to making them well. Like it or not, if you have come back from the brink, you have to be more aware and do more 'training' than the average person! It is like any skill that you lose when you stop practising it.

Before anyone rises up in anger, if a person has a recurrence, this does not mean they are responsible. All behavioural medicine does is increase the odds of wellness. It does not cause it or guarantee it.

At a lecture in Dublin some years ago, we heard Professor Anthony Clare say, 'Critical mass is essential in medicine.' Just as with antibiotics, critical mass is like practising the violin or learning a language. Nothing much seems to happen at first. The same applies in Behavioural Medicine. Your body is, or has been, going through trauma. Full recovery takes time.

~ SUMMARY ~

After 90 days of a comprehensive Behavioural Medicine programme, many patients feel so well that they stop doing what is making them well. This is risky!

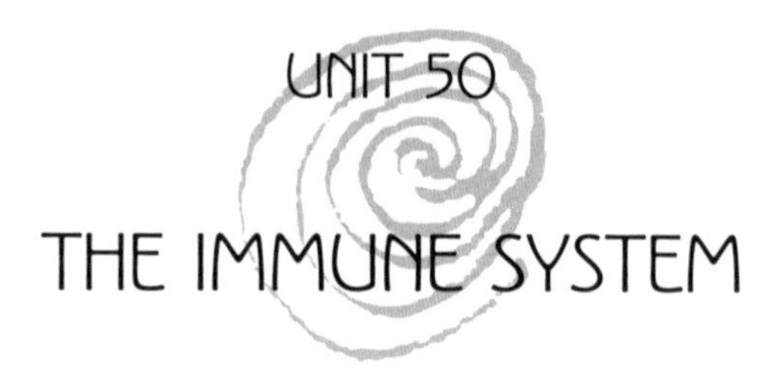

UNIT 50

THE IMMUNE SYSTEM

If our bodies are attacked by fungi, viruses, parasites, or bacteria, a complex reaction begins:

- Viruses try to replicate before the immune system can gear up.
- Macrophage cells recognise the threat and begin to engulf and destroy the attacker.
- Stimulated by the release of interleukins from macrophages, helper T cells and interferons (NK cells) join the attack on the infected cells. These also attack cancer cells.
- The Helper T cells (the battle managers of the immune system) send out signals to B cells and cytotoxic T cells to join the attack.
- B cells produced in the bones mature into plasma cells which, in turn, produce antibodies (memory).
- Antibodies are Y-shaped proteins designed to recognise a particular attacker or invader. They bind to the infected cells and neutralise them.
- Cytotoxic T cells wage chemical warfare on virally infected cells by firing lethal proteins at them.
- As the battle is won, Suppressor T cells help the immune system to gear down, as otherwise it might attack the body.
- As the invaders are defeated, the immune system creates memory T and B cells, ensuring that next time that the enemy will be recognised and beaten more swiftly.

An out of balance or suppressed immune response (resulting from stress, treatment etc.) will inhibit this magnificent system.

~ SUMMARY ~

The immune system is in the front line of our internal defence system with cancer. It can be helped using evidence-based methods.

PART 6

SOME USEFUL TECHNIQUES AND INTERVENTIONS

UNIT 51

STATE MANAGEMENT AND ANCHORING

An anchor or trigger is any stimulus that produces a consistent emotional or physical response pattern in a person. It is like a piece of human software in the brain that making an association between different things.

An anchor generally comes from connecting a stimulus to a strong emotion, which, with repetition, can cause conditioning. All of this happens at an unconscious level. Making these associations is what allows us to know what is enjoyable for us and what is not. Anchors can be either positive or negative. Examples of positive anchors might be: perfume, the smell of freshly baked bread, a particular piece of music or the sight of your home after a tiring day. Examples of negative anchors might be the sight of physical violence, the smell of a hospital, the sound of gritty chalk scraping down a blackboard or an expression on someone's face.

Numerous studies have shown that cancer patients will sometimes report feeling nauseous or distressed at even the smell of the hospital foyer, the sight of a particular medical person or the colour of a particular medication. The unconscious has made an automated connection between the stimulus (the smell of the foyer) and the response (feeling nauseous). This unpleasant anchored unconscious response may be resolved with help from a skilled therapist by creating a new response to the stimulus.

The following process from Neuro-Linguistic Programming (a form of Cognitive Behavioural Therapy) can enable you to create a reliable triggering mechanism to fire off positive resourceful states or feelings whenever you need them, without even having to think about it and, as importantly, to blow out the negative ones!

SIMPLE ANCHORING TECHNIQUE

Your objective is to develop the ability to create a positive resourceful state, on demand, by a simple physical gesture such as joining the thumb and little finger of your left hand together and inhaling sharply through the nose.

1. Make a short list of positive emotions, such as: excited, happy, calm, confident, resourceful, successful, etc. Select one such positive emotion from the list, and remember a specific event or time when you felt that emotion. Now identify what seemed like the peak moment in that situation.
2. As you recall that moment, and the good feelings that went with it, allow your eyes to close. Mentally, step back inside the memory as though you are right there, experiencing the good feelings (as best you can). As you experience them, join the thumb and little finger of your left hand together and inhale sharply through your nose (so you can hear it) almost as though you are inhaling the good feelings. Immediately release the finger, the breath, and the memory.
3. Now, select another time when you felt really good (happy, confident, pleased, successful etc.) and again, identify the peak moment in that situation.
4. Repeat Step 2.
5. Finally select a third time when you felt really good (happy, confident, pleased, successful etc.) and again, identify the peak moment in that situation.
6. Repeat Step 2.

Note: This exercise should take a maximum of five minutes daily. Remember, you are seeking to build up a powerful anchor, so repeating this exercise on a daily basis, for a couple of weeks, will enable you to develop a new skill!

KEYS TO SUCCESSFUL ANCHORING

- Make sure you connect strong positive feelings to your resource anchor. Wishy-washy feelings will give you a wishy-washy anchor.
- Timing - Join the thumb and little finger and inhale at the peak of the remembered good experience.
- Make sure you apply the same degree of pressure each time that you join the thumb and little finger.
- Anchoring ensures always having access to your greatest resources or strengths! Much of human behaviour consists of unconscious pre-programmed responses. We are constantly anchoring; it's impossible

not to! If anchors don't support or enable you, change or replace them with a new stimulus/response. Anchoring is neurological linking at the peak of an emotional response.

- The power or impact of an anchor is in direct ratio to the intensity of the emotion(s) to which it is attached. For an anchor to be effective, when the stimulus is triggered, the person must be in a fully connected state (in the picture, seeing things through their own eyes), with the whole body involved! Anchors do not need lengthy conditioning. When a person is health-challenged, a positive anchoring method is a very method for managing how you feel.
- Once you have practiced this anchoring exercise for about two weeks, whenever you feel in need of an emotional or physical boost, just join your thumb and little finger together and inhale sharply and you will be able to access feelings of resourcefulness on demand. Also, whenever you experience a positive emotion or feeling in your day to day life, you can add this onto your anchor to strengthen it further by joining thumb and little finger and inhaling sharply.
- Do have fun in learning this process! Like any new skill, practice it before attempting to use it.

~ SUMMARY ~

Anchoring means being able to change the way you feel whenever you want.

KEY NOTES

UNIT 52

RULE OF 6 – COGNITIVE RESTRUCTURING/REFRAMING

The Rule of 6 technique comes from the North American Indian traditional wisdom. During the education of a young person, they were challenged by an elder to find six different yet credible ways of looking at a problem they were dealing with. This forced the young person to examine a problem from a range of different perspectives and enhanced their ability to deal with life challenges.

An example of this might be: 'My horse has dropped dead.'

1. This is a catastrophe I'll never get over this!
2. Why did the Gods pick on me? Why me?
3. I might have broken my neck if I had been riding him at the time! Whew!
4. My horse needed to be cared for. I'll look after the next one better!
5. This is an opportunity to get a better horse!
6. I was selfish with my horse. Maybe if I had shared it, somebody would be loaning me their horse now!

In the context of being diagnosed with a life threatening or quality-of-life threatening illness, patients have given these examples of diverse perspectives:

- Life is cruel to me! Why me?
- This 'disaster' has given me a chance to re-appraise my life!
- I can now focus on my needs and priorities.
- I now value each and every day and enjoy a far higher quality of life.
- I have not been caring for myself – until now. I can change that!
- Being ill has enabled me to meet a lot of genuine sincere people!

The objective of the exercise is to free up psychological ways of looking at an event. A patient who dwells exclusively on the extreme negative will tend to have a lower immune function than a person who sees all the perspectives.

~ SUMMARY ~

Multiple ways of looking at life-events remove blocks to healing.

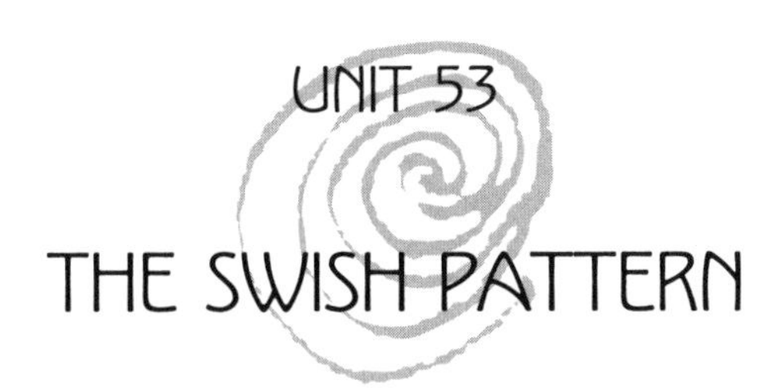

UNIT 53
THE SWISH PATTERN

Developed by Dr. Richard Bandler and Dr John Grinder back in the 1970s, the Swish Pattern is used for changing any habitual way of thinking or behaving. If certain situations tend to trigger you into unresourceful mental states or behaviours you don't want, this is a simple yet highly effective to turn off the auto-pilot in the unconscious which provides reactions or responses and to introduce a more desired response.

THE PROCESS

Step 1. In your mind, create a picture or image of a habit, behaviour pattern or situation that you want to change (perhaps where you are stuck!). See, through your own eyes, what is going on when this situation occurs. This is Picture No. 1.

Step 2. Now, in your mind, create a disassociated image (seeing yourself as part of the picture) of how you wish to behave or react differently. See the person you wish to become or the outcome you want, e.g. tumour to shrink; or wound to heal (vividly and in detail). This is Picture No. 2.

Step 3. Now, in your mind, place Picture No. 1, large and bright, on an imaginary screen in front of you and in the lower right hand corner of this image, place a small dark version of Picture No. 2.

Step 4. Now, abruptly, have Picture No. 2 break through and totally obliterate Picture No. 1. Now Picture No. 2 is large, bright and attractive, while picture No. 1 shrinks down to bottom right. Then immediately let the images go and open your eyes.

Speed is of the essence. Make sure the old image fades at exactly the same time as the new one explodes onto the stage of your inner mind. It can help this technique if you accompany the changeover by an internal or external 'swish' sound. You must see and feel that small dark Picture No. 2 suddenly become huge and bright and explode through Picture No. 1, destroying it and replacing it.

Step 5. Repeat the process a minimum of five times with each project and enjoy the results. You are re-conditioning habitual ways of thinking

~ SUMMARY ~

Unhelpful automated reactions and responses can be reprogrammed.

KEY NOTES

'I really enjoyed the programme. I still use some of the techniques and exercises we learned. The emphasis on being positive and proactive about one's health stayed with me.' *M.D., Co. Louth*

UNIT 54

A QI GONG METHOD FOR STRESS MANAGEMENT

Qi Gong is an ancient Chinese method of energy medicine which focuses on the art and practice of moving Qi (life energy) in the body for healing purposes.

THE PROCES

1. Sit on the front edge of a straight-backed chair. Place your feet flat on the ground, shoulder-width apart – use a cushion under them if necessary.
2. Hold the spine straight, but not rigid. Hold the head level with the back of the neck elongated, chin level with the floor.
3. Soften the shoulders down and outwards and let your hands rest lightly on your knees, palms facing upwards.
4. Relax the chest.
5. Breathe softly and slowly through the nose, creating an awareness of the breath coming into an imaginary point in the centre of the chest. Feel this breath sinking from the chest down to the lower abdomen, and continue this feeling with each outward breath. Whilst continuing to breathe softly, become aware of your breath travelling between the chest and lower abdomen. Get a feeling of all the tension in your neck and shoulders flowing down your arms and out through your upturned palms.
6. At first, take at least five minutes – or more if it's comfortable for you. (As you become used to this practice, you can do it for 20 minutes or more each day.)
7. To finish the session, take your hands (palms still facing upwards, as though gathering energy from the air), out to your sides and over your head, fingers not quite touching. Then continue the movement of the hands down in front of the face, bringing the energy down in front of your body to lower abdomen. Rest your hand on the lower abdomen, one hand on top of the other.
8. Hold the final position for a few moments to experience the energy.

Adapted by Gary Collins, TCM Practitioner, specialising in Qi Gong and T'ai Chi Chuan

~ SUMMARY ~

Qi Gong breathing stimulates 'life force' in the body.

KEY NOTES

'I would say that the programme was really fantastic, that it gave me incredible strength to get through all my treatment, and that it has had a long-lasting positive effect on my life. It definitely played a huge part in my recovery and it was empowering above all – and I am grateful to have taken part in it.' *H.M., Co. Wicklow*

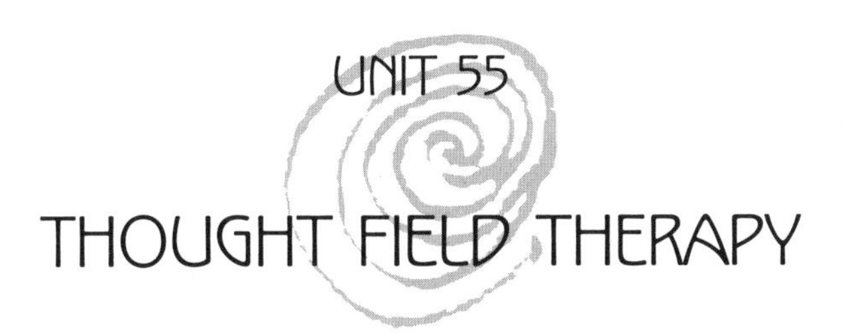

UNIT 55

THOUGHT FIELD THERAPY

The one common factor among people dealing with serious illness of all types and stages is anxiety. People who are waiting for the results of tests or biopsies are frequently in a highly anxious state. The first indications that something is not right can produce a degree of anxiety, but there is something about hearing the diagnosis confirmed by a consultant that people describe as 'traumatic'.

Even when several months have elapsed, and the offending tumour removed or the arterial blockage bypassed, the anticipation of a routine quarterly check-up with the consultant can be a daunting experience. Even the prospect of an imminent GP's appointment may be stressful. Unfortunately there is little support for patients coping with this added anxiety.

You might say it is perfectly normal and natural to be anxious at a time like this – and of course it is. However, if this period of anxiety is prolonged, it can affect the immune system at a time when it most needs to be working optimally. The list of physical and psychological effects of sustained stress is quite extensive, causing a hormonal imbalance which is likely to interfere with the body's natural healing ability. In particular, it may affect a patient's ability to get adequate sleep which is essential in restoring equilibrium to mind and body.

Over the last four years we (SC and RD) have been using a very effective technique for resolving anxiety and trauma (amongst many other psychological conditions). It was developed by Roger Callahan, Ph.D., a clinical psychologist in the USA who had been working mainly with cognitive (thinking) forms of psychotherapy since 1950. In the early 1980s, by adapting procedures from other disciplines, including chiropractic and acupressure, Dr. Callahan devised a process that could eliminate many psychological problems. After more than 20 years of extensive research, he has produced a user-friendly method that can be used by anyone to alleviate anxiety or distress. As we go to press, patients in the USA are also reporting success in using Thought Field Therapy (TFT) to eliminate many of the side-effects of cancer treatment.

THE PROCESS

At the most basic level, a patient can be taught a simple method of tapping with the fingers on particular pressure points on the body, while holding a specific negative emotion or distressing thought in mind.

The objective is not only to significantly reduce the level of distress, but also to eliminate it completely – which, amazingly, it does in the majority of cases.

Roger Callahan's techniques are so successful, that they have spawned a number of imitations on which much has been written in the last few years. Needless to say, the best way to learn this process is from a certified Thought Field Therapy practitioner – and, fortunately, they are now within reach in most parts of the World. You can find one through the official TFT website, www.tftrx.com. However, if you can't find someone within reach, there are books available which explain the technique – Dr. Callahan's most recent publication is *Tapping the Healer Within*, published by Piatkus Press in the UK.

~ SUMMARY ~

Anxiety depresses the immune system.
Unhelpful anxiety can be easily cleared.

KEY NOTES

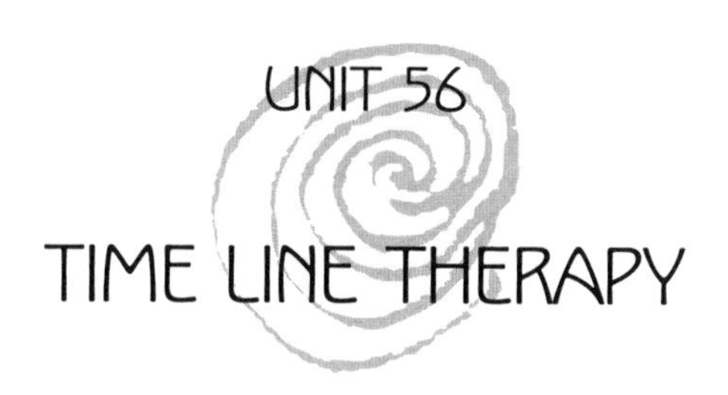

UNIT 56

TIME LINE THERAPY

Neuro-Linguistic Programming (NLP) is a form of cognitive behavioural therapy which emerged in the 1970s in California. NLP spawned a set of psychological techniques which enable clients to bring about rapid changes in unwanted reactions, responses and behaviours.

Tad James, M.S., Ph.D., developed a basic concept in NLP, that our experience of the world and, indeed, our personalities, are influenced by our concept of time and the way that we store both remembered and forgotten significant emotional events from the past.

What can happens is that the negative emotional memory from the first event, when this emotion was first experienced, sets us up to experiencing the feelings from that event in all subsequent events involving this emotion. With the passage of time, following on a number of similar events, a pattern (or gestalt) of emotions is built up. A relatively minor event in today can trigger or re-activate a flood of emotional from past events. Anger, sadness, fear, hurt, or guilt, are the major emotions on which such patterns are built. Road rage would be an example of where there is a disproportionate emotional response to a minor event in today.

Time Line Therapy is a gentle, yet powerful, way of releasing the trapped emotional energy from significant past negative memories and yet, at the same time, preserving what was to be learned from these incidents. In this way, old memories have no longer the power to evoke distressing emotions.

Dr. Tad James and Wyatt *Time Line Therapy and the Basis of Personality,* Woodsmall, Meta Publications, (1988)

~ SUMMARY ~

We do not have to be at the mercy of our past negative emotions.
They can be easily healed and released.

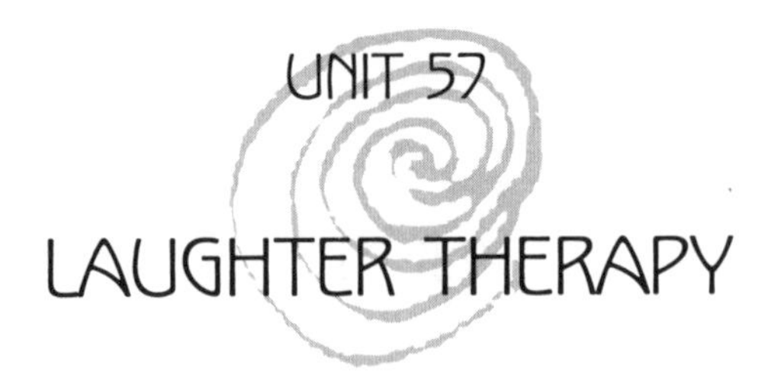

UNIT 57

LAUGHTER THERAPY

'A merry heart does good like a medicine,
but a broken spirit dries the bones.'
PROVERBS 17:22

Norman Cousins, former editor of the *Saturday Review*, brought the attention of the medical community to the possibility that laughter may have a healing potential. In 1964, he was diagnosed with ankylosing spondylitis, a progressive degenerative disease of the collagen tissue. His physicians gave him little hope for recovery, indicating that a possible cause of his illness was heavy-metal poisoning. From reading Hans Selye's book, *The Stress of life,* Cousins recalled that research showed that negative emotions could create chemical changes in the body that could, eventually, lead to adrenal exhaustion. He suspected that positive emotions might create changes in the body that would enhance or accelerate his recovery process.

Since the behaviour of laughter tends to open a person to emotions of joy and hope, Cousins began viewing funny films to stimulate deep belly laughter. After each laughing episode, he noticed that he could sleep more comfortably without the need for analgesia or sedation. He also discovered that laughter stimulated a decrease in his sedimentation rate, indicating a reversal of the inflammatory response. After his recovery, Cousins was appointed an adjunct professor at UCLA Medical School where he led research into the beneficial effects of laughter.

Clinical research is now demonstrating clearly that humour and laughter in our lives can significantly enhance the effectiveness of the immune system. Illness, either acute onset or chronic, is generally a stressful event. Hospitalisation, separation from family, invasive procedures, complex technology or unfamiliar caregivers, all can create feelings of anxiety, loneliness, discomfort, anger, panic, and depression for patients. These emotions are now known to produce physiological changes that interfere with the body's natural 'fight back' mechanisms at the precise time when these need to be boosted. Humour and laughter can reverse this.

Humour is a perceptual process that is processed in the mind, whereas laughter is a behavioural response, it happens in the body!

INTERESTING THOUGHTS ON LAUGHTER

- Laughter has been proven to provide an effective counterbalance to stress, helplessness and depression.
- Laughter is sometimes hard to start – but only at first.
- Laughter creates powerful biochemical changes that help the body.
- Caregivers need to laugh too. Researchers have also shown that putting a smile on your face, even if you are not happy, also triggers helpful hormones.
- Clinical research shows the following benefits of laughter:
  - Serum cortisol level decrease (enhances immune response).
  - The baseline of adrenalin decreases (enhances immune response).
  - Increase in natural killer (NK) cell numbers and activity (NK cells attack cancer cells).
  - Increase in numbers of helper-T cells (better immune function).
  - Salivary immunoglobulin A (IgA) level increase (our first line defence against infections).
- Try the following:
  - Watch funny movies, videos, or films on TV
  - Actively seek out positive good humoured and funny people
  - Look for things to laugh at in everyday life
  - Avoid negative people
  - Give yourself permission to laugh

Cousins, N., *Anatomy of an Illness.* New York, Norton and Co (1979)
Cousins, N., *Head First – The Biology of Hope.* New York, Dutton (1989)

~ SUMMARY ~

Humour and laughter release 'happy' hormones and boost immune function.

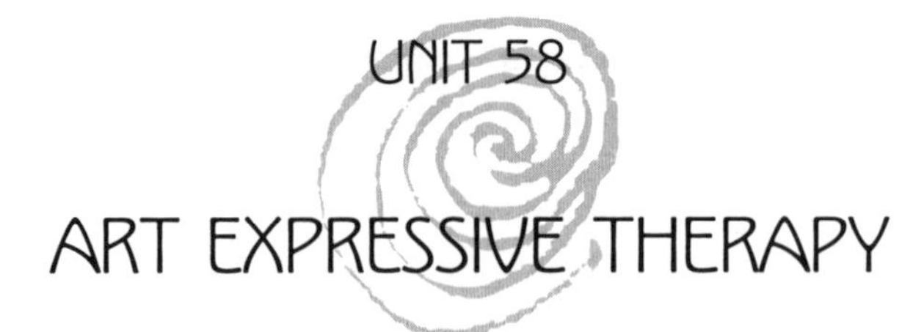

UNIT 58

ART EXPRESSIVE THERAPY

THE PROCESS

- Art Therapy gains access to feelings and emotions that are too difficult to express.
- It gives opportunity for self-expression, building of confidence and a sense of autonomy.
- It can be used as a tool to gain insight into one's feelings of anxiety, loss and isolation.
- It can provide an opportunity for people to rediscover their capacity for spontaneity and creativity at difficult times in their lives.
- Art Therapy is particularly valuable for people who are experiencing serious illness.

~ SUMMARY ~

Music, movement and dance therapies provide similar means of expressing emotion, and boosting self-healing.

KEY NOTES

UNIT 59

EVALUATING ALTERNATIVE AND COMPLEMENTARY THERAPIES

The following checklist is for consideration by anyone facing a life-threatening or 'quality of life'-threatening condition. This emerged from the reading of over 500 books in the area and more than 2,000 research papers. Potential sources of stress are listed, as well as sources of healing - these are sometimes interchangeable!

Having completed the twelve-week basic programme, you are here provided with an immediate check-list with which to brain-storm other areas for potential investigation with your 'important other' or health crisis counsellor. Many of the therapies listed here are untried and controversial so it is important to consider the following questions when considering any 'alternative' or complementary therapy.

CHECKLIST

- Has research been done on this therapy?
- Is there at least strong suggestive evidence that it works?
- Does it hurt?
- What are the side effects?
- Do I know anyone who has used it?
- What did they think about it?
- Will my doctor support me?
- Is it viewed as dangerous by the medical profession?
- Could it interfere with my current treatment?
- Can I trust the practitioner?
- What books have been written on it?
- How is it rated by guides to complementary therapies, such as *Health Which*?
- Is there a national organisation of practitioners?
- Is the practitioner a member in good standing of a national organisation?
- Is the practitioner insured?
- What will it cost?

- What is the time commitment (for therapy sessions/my own daily practice)?
- What is the energy commitment?

~ SUMMARY ~

There are many alternative and complementary therapies out there but they all must be evaluated so as first to do no harm.

KEY NOTES

SUMMARY

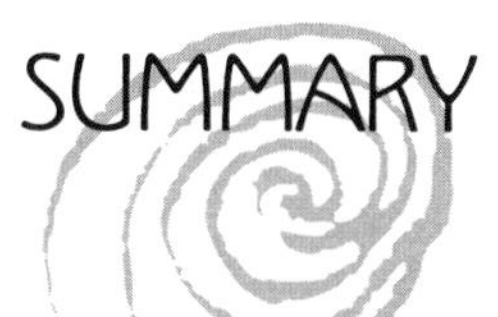

This book is for patients diagnosed with some life-threatening or 'quality of life'-threatening condition, to enable them make a comprehensive and well-formed choice as to their response. It draws on more than 50 years of research in behavioural medicine or psychoneuroimmunology (PNI) from more than 40 universities around the world, combined with the experience of the authors in eight years of clinical research.

The principles and methods outlined suggest that if patients engage in a comprehensive and timely 90-day Behavioural Medicine programme, they can significantly increase the odds of admission in to the 'winners circle' of those who recover.

There is no single cause of cancer or heart disease. These chronic diseases have been shown to have multiple co-factors in terms of causality combined with the passage of time; their resolution is unlikely to be significantly different. We are both the custodians of evolution and the experiments in evolution

This book has tried to identify many of the co-factors that have been shown to contribute to the worsening of a disease process as well as the co-factors that have been shown to contribute to improvement or recovery. In the light of the available research, to withhold a comprehensive Behavioural Medicine programme as an option in the treatment of cancer is tantamount to abuse.

Fourteen years after Spiegel, we still have virtually nothing. Eleven years after Ornish, we still have virtually nothing. If we wait for research, it will be another fifty years before we have data, let alone clinical applications – in the meantime, millions will die.

In the 1840s Hungarian-born obstetrician Dr. Ignaz Semmelweiss showed the death rate of newborn infants and mothers decreased to almost zero when obstetricians learned to wash or sterilise their hands. This pioneer of anti-sepsis in obstetrics died in an institution, insane, after many years fighting the system, fighting the orthodox medical profession, completely disillusioned by its professed ideals. After some sham trials, they went back to their old practices. It is estimated that during those years, almost one million women died unnecessarily, waiting for antisepsis to be accepted. It was almost twenty years later, in the 1860s, that University of Glasgow surgery professor, Joseph Lister, was knighted for finally introducing anti-sepsis.

Psychosocial behavioural medicine been shown, albeit in fragments, to have a similar potential to greatly enhance the prospects of survival amongst those suffering with life threatening and major quality-of-life conditions.

'Mankind is annoyed because the truth is so simple' Goethe.

To become an expert mountaineer, you have to study and emulate what other top mountaineers have done – and you may still die on the mountain!

APPENDIX 1 - IMMUNE BOOSTERS

- A pet
- Balance in life
- Beliefs (positive)
- Breath work (diaphragmatic)
- Calorie restriction
- Connectedness
- Crying
- Emotion expression
- Exercise (aerobic AND anaerobic)
- Foods rich in antioxidants and EFAs
- Foods (low fat/unsaturated fats/high fibre)
- Forgiveness
- Herbs (Shitake mushrooms, Reishi Mushrooms, Garlic, Echinacea, Essiac)
- Tea (Ginseng, Astralagus, Green and Black Tea, Ginger)
- Journalling
- Laughter/fun
- Massage (caution – check with your doctors)
- Meditation
- Optimism
- Relaxation training/conditioning
- Sense of control
- Social support/community/intimacy
- Vitamins and minerals (antioxidants)
- Yoga

~ SUMMARY ~

There is a wide range of things you the patient can do yourself support your immune system and boost self-healing.

APPENDIX 2 - IMMUNE SUPPRESSORS

- Ageing (mental/physical)
- Anger/resentment (repressed)
- Antibiotics (some)
- Being too passive or too aggressive
- Beliefs and Attitudes (negative)
- Chemotherapy (frequently but not always)
- Depression (chronic)
- Diet (high fat/saturated fats)
- Disease (chronic – low grade)
- Emotion suppression (including historical)
- Excessive caffeine
- Helpless/hopeless (chronic)
- Many medications
- Negativity (chronic)
- Over-nutrition
- Perfectionism
- Pollution (including noise)
- Radiotherapy
- Recreational drugs
- Relationship difficulties (chronic)
- Sedentary lifestyle (chronic)
- Sense of loss of control
- Sleep disorders
- Smoking
- Stress (chronic/excessive)
- Sugars (excessive)
- Surgery
- Time pressured (chronic)
- Unhappiness

~ SUMMARY ~

There are multiple suppressors of immune function which you can correct.

APPENDIX 3 - HEALTH CRISIS COUNSELLORS

Teresa McSwiney
Derry, Northern Ireland
Tel: 02871 265 849

Dr. Sean Collins
Donnybrook, Dublin 4
Tel: 01 260 0118 &
Bantry, Co. Cork
Tel: 028 32946

Mary Langton
Blackrock, Co. Dublin
Tel: 01 278 3624

Rhoda Draper
Donnybrook, Dublin 4
Tel: 01 260 0118

Billey Ryan
Glenageary, Co. Dublin
Tel: 01 214 5891

Dr. Aine Abbott
Derry, Northern Ireland
Tel: 02871 358 336

Brian Hennessy
Merrion Square, Dublin 2
Tel: 087 257 6935

Olivia Nally
Donnybrook, Dublin 4 &
Phibsboro', Dublin 7
Tel: 01 831 8104

Bridget Greaney
Lucan, Co. Dublin
Tel: 01 628 1012

Patricia Swann
Donegal & Derry
Tel: 074 91 38457

Graham Egan
Navan Road, Dublin 7
Tel: 838 7241

Sherrie Scott-Keegan
Donegal
Tel: 071 985 2925

APPENDIX 4 - CONTACTS, ORGANISATIONS, RESOURCES AND WEBSITES

Arc Cancer Support Centre
Arc House
65 Eccles Street, Dublin 7
Tel: 01 830 7333
www.arccancersupport.ie

Ardagh Clinic
118 Stillorgan Road
Dublin 4
Tel: 01 260 0115
e-mail: ardaghclinic@eircom.net
www.wellness-recovery.com

Christian Meditation Centre
4 Eblana Avenue
Dun Laoghaire, Co. Dublin
Tel: 01 280 1505
e-mail:maranatha@wccmireland.org
www.wccmireland.org

Derry Well Woman
17 Queen Street
Derry
Northern Ireland
Tel: 00 44 287 1360 777

The Psycho-Oncology Units
St. James's Hospital and
St. Vincent's University Hospital
Dublin

Irish Association for Counselling & Psychotherapy
8 Cumberland Street
Dun Laoghaire, Co. Dublin
Tel: 01 230 0061
iacp@irish-counselling.ie
www.irish-counselling.ie

Irish Council for Psychotherapy
73 Quinn's Road
Shankill, Co. Dublin
Tel: 272 2105
e-mail: info@icpty.ie
www.icpty.ie

Irish Cancer Society
5 Northumberland Road
Dublin 4
Tel: 01 231 0500
Freefone: 1800 200 700
e-mail: reception@irishcancer.ie
www.cancer.ie

Bristol Cancer Help Centre
Cornwallis Grove
Bristol BS8 4PG, UK
Tel: +44 117 980 9500
e-mail: info@bristolcancerhelp.org
www.bristolcancerhelp.org

The Irish Institute of Counselling and Hypnotherapy Tel: 01 2600115

Irish Institute of Counselling & Hypnotherapy
6 Nutley Lane
Dublin 4
Tel: 01 260 0115
iich@eircom.net

Irish Yoga Association
Pallas Park, Blueball
Tullamore, Co. Offaly
Tel: (0)506 54880
e-mail: iya@eircom.net
www.homepage.eircom.net/~iya

Samaritans
112 Marlborough Street
Dublin 1
Tel: 01 872 7700
Callsave: 1850 609 090

Slánú Cancer Help Centre,
Birchhall, Oughterard,
Co.Galway.
Tel: 091 550050
e-mail: info@slanu.ie
www.slanu.ie

Yoga Therapy Ireland
20 Auburn Drive,
Killiney, Co. Dublin.
Tel/Fax: 01 2352120.
e-mail : yti@eircom.net
www.yogatherapyireland.com

The Breath & Stress Clinic
Attn: Michael Comyn
Ardee, Dublin, Belfast
Tel: 1890 2000 47
e-mail: michael@breathandstress.com
www.breathandstress.com

Dublin Meditation Centre (Buddhist)
42 Lr. Leeson Street, Dublin 2
Tel: 01 661 5934
e-mail:
info@dublinmeditationcentre.org
www.dublinmeditationcentre.org

APPENDIX 5 - WEBSITES AND BOOKS

Arc Cancer Support Centre www.arccancersupport.ie
Ardagh Clinic www.wellness-recovery.com
Dr. Ralph Moss's website www.cancerdecisions.com
Irish Cancer Society www.cancer.ie
Irish Institute of Counselling & Hypnotherapy www.iich.ie
Slánú Cancer Help Centre www.slanu.ie
Yoga Therapy Ireland www.yogatherapyireland.com
VHI www.vhihealthe.com
BUPA www.bupaireland.ie
Life Extension Organisation www.lef.org
American Cancer Society www.cancer.org

You will find a great number of books in the bibliography, in fact between us we have read over 2,000 books on the topic of health. On this page we have picked out some books you might like to keep within reach and use as a reference.

Ralph W. Moss, PhD,
Antioxidants against Cancer, Equinox (2000)

Patrick Quillan, PhD,
Beating Cancer with Nutrition, Nutrition Times Press (2nd Ed. 2001)

Earl Mindell, (2002)
Food as Medicine: What You Can Eat to Help Prevent Everything from Colds to Heart Disease to Cancer Pocket Books (2nd Ed. 2001)

Earl Mindell,
Earl Mindell's New Vitamin Bible: 25th Anniversary Edition, Warner Books (2004)

Peter J. D'Adamo, PhD,
Eat Right for Your Type, Century Books (2001)

Udo Erasmus, PhD
Fats that Heal, Fats that Kill, Alive Books (1998)

Greg Anderson
50 Essential Things to Do when the Doctors says IT'S CANCER, G.P. Putnam's Sons (1993)

BIBLIOGRAPHY

Anderson, G. (1993) *50 Essential Things To Do When the Doctor says It's Cancer*. New York: Penguin.
Andreas, S. and Andreas, C. (1987) *Change Your Mind, and Keep the Change*. Utah: Real People Press.
Bach, R. (1972). *Jonathan Livingston Seagull*. London: Turnstone.
Benson, H.(1996) *Timeless Healing*. New York: Simon and Schuster.
Benson, H. (1975) *The Relaxation Response*. New York: Avon Books.
Benson, H. (1984) *Beyond the Relaxation Response*. New York: Berkeley Books.
Benson, H. (1987) *Your Maximum Mind.* New York: Avon Books.
Benson, H., and Stuart, E. (1992) *The Wellness Book*. New York: Simon and Schuster
Borysenko, J. (1990) *Guilt is the Teacher, Love is the Lesson.* New York: Warner Books
Borysenko, J. (1994) *The Power of the Mind to Heal*. Enfield: Grove Publications.
Brigham, D. Davis (1994) *Imagery for Getting Well – Clinical Applications of Behavioural Medicine.* New York: Norton.
Brody, H. (2000) *The Placebo Response*. New York: Harper Collins.
Brohn, P. (1987) *The Bristol Programme*. London: Century.
Brown, D. and Fromm, E. (1987) *Hypnosis and Behavioural Medicine.* London: Erlbaum.
Buckman, R. (1996) *What You Really Need to Know About Cancer*. London: Macmillan.
Burns, D.D. (1990) *The Feeling Good Handbook.* New York: Plume.
Callahan, R.J. (2001) *Tapping the Healer Within*. Chicago: Contemporary Books.
Cameron, E. and Pauling, L. (1979) *Cancer and Vitamin C.* Philadelphia: Camino Books.
Chopra, D. (1987) *Creating Health.* London: Grafton.
Chopra, D. (1989) *Quantum Healing*. New York: Bantam.
Chopra, D. (1990) *Perfect Health.* New York: Bantam.
Cohen, K. (1997) *The Way of Qigong.* New York: Ballantine.
Conduit, Ed. (1995) *The Body Under Stress.* Hove: Erlbaum.

Cornelius, R. R. (1996) *The Science of Emotion*. New Jersey: Prentice-Hall.

Cousins, N. (1979) *Anatomy of an Illness*. London: Bantam Books.

Cousins, N. (1989) *Head First, The Biology of Hope.* New York: Dutton.

Cousins, N. (1983) *The Healing Heart.* New York: Norton.

Diamond, J.(1998) *Because Cowards Get Cancer too*. London: Vermilion.

Diamond, J. (2001). *Snake Oil*, Surrey: Vintage.

Dilts, R., Hallbom, T., and Smith, S. (1990) *Beliefs, Pathways to Health and Well-being*. Oregon: Metamorphous.

Dossey, L. (1991) *Healing Break-throughs*. London: Piatkus.

Dossey, L. (1993) *Healing Words*. New York: Harper-Collins.

Dreher, H. (1995) *The Immune Power Personality.* London: Penguin.

Dubovsky, S. L. (1997) *Mind Body Deceptions*. London: Norton

Dworkis, S.(1997) *Recovery Yoga.* New York: Three Rivers Press.

Erasmus, U. (1986) *Fats that Heal, Fats that Kill*. Burnaby BC: Alive Books.

Frahm, A. E., and Frahm, D. J. (1992) *A Cancer Battle Plan.* Colorado: Pinon Press.

Frankl, V. E. (1963) *Man's Search for Meaning*. New York: Washington Square Press.

Frantz, R. and Pattakos, A.N. (1996) *Intuition at Work, Pathways to Unlimited Possibilities*. San Francisco: Sterling and Stone.

Friedman, H. S. (1992) *The Self-Healing Personality*. New York: Plume.

Fudlder, S. (1996) *The Handbook of Alternative and Complementary Medicine*. Oxford: OUP.

Galland, L. (1997) *Power Healing*. New York: Random House.

Gawler, I. (1984) *You Can Conquer Cancer*. Melbourne: Hill of Content.

Gillis, J. (1995) *The Heart Attack Prevention and Recovery Handbook*. Vancouver: Hartley and Marks.

Golan, R., M.D., (1995) *Optimal Wellness*, New York: Ballentine

Goleman, D. and Gurin, J. (1993) *Mind/Body Medicine, How to Use Your Mind for Better Health*. New York: Spectrum America.

Goleman, D. (1993) *Mind Body Medicine*. New York: Consumer Report Books.

Goleman, D. (1996) *Emotional Intelligence*. London: Bloomsbury.
Goleman, D. (1998) *The Meditative Mind*. New York: Putnam Books.
Gordon, N.F. and Gibbons, L.W. (1990) *The Cooper Clinic Cardiac Rehabilitation Program*. New York: Simon and Schuster.
Hersh, S.P. (1986) *Beyond Miracles – Living with Cancer*. Chicago: Contemporary Books.
Hilgard, E.R. and Hilgard, J.R. (1975) *Hypnosis in the Relief of Pain*. California: Kaufmann.
Hirshberg, C. and Barasch, M.I, (1995) *Remarkable Recovery*. London: Headline.
James, T. (1989) *The Secret of Creating Your Future*. Honolulu: Advanced Neuro Dynamics.
Jones, E. and Morris, A. (1998) *Cell Biology and Genetics*. London: Mosby.
Kabat-Zinn, J. (1991) *Full Catastrophe Living*. New York: Dell.
Kearney, M. (1996) *Mortally Wounded*. Cork: Marino Books.
King, P. (1994) *Quest for Life*. California: Dawn Publications.
Kirsta, A. (1986) *The Book of Stress Survival*. London, Simon and Schuster.
Koestler, A. (1967) *The Ghost in the Machine*. New York: Macmillan Company.
Kubler-Ross, E. (1970) *On Death and Dying*. London: Tavistock/Routledge.
Laskow, L. (1992) *Healing with Love*. San Francisco: Harper.
Lerner, M. (1994) *Choices in Healing*. Cambridge, Massachusetts: MIT Press.
LeShan, L. (1974) *How to Meditate*. London: Thorsons.
LeShan, L. (1977) *You Can Fight For Your Life*. New York: Evans.
Levine, B. H. (1991) *Your Body Believes Every Word You Say*. California: Aslan.
Lynn, J. (1992) *Cancer Treatment and Care*. Plymouth: Northcote House.
Maltz, M. (1960) *Psycho-Cybernetics*. California: Wiltshire Book Co.
Markham, U. (1993) *Living with Change*. Dorset: Element Books.
Martin, P. (1997) *The Sickening Mind*. London: Harper Collins.
McDermott, I, and O'Connor, J. (1996) *NLP and Health*. London: Thorsons.

McWilliams, J. R and McWilliams, P. (1988) *You Can't Afford the Luxury of a Negative Thought.* Los Angeles: Prelude.

Meek, J. (1990) *Immune Power.* London: MacDonald.

Meek, J., and Holford, P. (1998) *Boost Your Immune System.* London: Piatkus.

Mindell, E. (1994) *The Food Medicine Bible.* London: Souvenir.

Moyers, B. (1993) *Healing and the Mind.* New York: Doubleday.

Nadel, L. (2001) *Dancing with the Wind.* New York: Paraview Press.

Nuland, S.B. (1997) *The Wisdom of the Body.* London: Chatto and Windus.

O'Donohue, J. (1997) *Anam Cara – Spiritual Wisdom from the Celtic World.* London: Bantam.

Ornish, D. (1982) *Stress, Diet and your Heart.* New York: Signet.

Ornish, D. (1990) *Dr. Dean Ornish's Programme for Reversing Heart Disease.* New York: Century.

Page, C. R. (1992) *Frontiers of Health.* Essex: Daniel.

Patel, C. (1994) *Fighting Heart Disease.* London: Dorling Kindersley.

Pelletier, K. R. (1992) *Mind as Healer, Mind as Slayer.* New York: Dell.

Pert, C. B. (1997) *Molecules of Emotion.* New York: Scribner

Puri, B. & Boyd, H. (2004) *The Natural Way to Beat Depression.* London: Hodder and Stoughton.

Robbins, A. (1992) *Awaken the Giant Within.* London: Simon and Schuster.

Rosenberg, S.A., and Barry, J. M. (1992) *The Transformed Cell.* London: Butler and Tanner.

Rossi, E. L., and Cheek, D. B. (1994) *Mind Body Therapy.* London: Norton

Rossi, E. L. (1986) *The Psychobiology of Mind-Body Healing.* New York: Norton.

Rossi, E. L. (1996) *The Symptom Path to Enlightenment.* California: Palisades Gateway.

Servan-Schreiber, D. (2004) *Healing without Freud or Prozac.* London: Rhodale

Shealy, C. (1995) *Miracles Do Happen.* Brisbane: Element Books.

Siegel, B. S. (1986) *Love, Medicine and Miracles.* London: Harper and Row.

Siegel, B. S. (1990) *Peace, Love and Healing.* London: Arrow.

Siegel, B. S. (1993) *Living, Loving and Healing.* London: Aquarian Press.

Sikora, K., and Thomas, H. (1989) *Fight Cancer.* London: BBC Books.

Simon, D. (1997) *The Wisdom of Healing.* New York: Harmony Books.

Simonton, O. C., and Matthews-Simonton, S. (1978) *Getting Well Again.* New York: Bantam.

Sinatra, S. (1996) *Heartbreak and Heart Disease.* Connecticut: Keats.

Skrabanek, P., and McCormick, J. (1992) *Follies and Fallacies in Medicine.* Glasgow: Tarragon.

Spiegel, D. (1993) *Living Beyond Limits.* New York: Times Books.

Spiegel, H. and Spiegel, D. (1978) *Trance and Treatment.* New York: American Psychiatric Press.

Stoll, A. (2001) *The Omega-3 Connection.* London: Simon & Schuster/Viacom.

Temoshok, L., and Dreher, H. (1993) *The Type C Connection.* New York: Penguin.

Thomas, H. and Sikora, K. (1995) *Cancer – A Positive Approach.* California: Thorsons.

Tobias, J. (1995) *Cancer – What every patient needs to know.* London: Bloomsbury.

Watkins, A. (1997) *Mind-Body Medicine.* Edinburgh: Livingstone.

Watts, G. (1992) *Pleasing the Patient.* London: Faber and Faber.

Weil, A. (1995) *Natural Health, Natural Medicine.* New York: Warner.

Weil, A. (1995) *Spontaneous Healing.* London: Warner.

Weil, A. (1997) *Eight Weeks to Optimum Health.* London: Warner.

Whittaker, J. (1985) *Reversing Heart Disease.* New York: Warner.

Winawer, S., and Shike, M. (1994) *Cancer Free.* London: Simon and Schuster.

Wollams, C. (2002) *Everything You Need To Know to Help You Beat Cancer.* Buckingham: Health Issues Ltd.

BIOGRAPHICAL INFORMATION

DR SEAN COLLINS is a counsellor and psychotherapist in private practice in Co. Dublin and Co. Cork, specialising in stress-related conditions with a particular emphasis on clinical applications of Behavioural Medicine.

Educated in Scoil Mhuire (CBS), Marino, Belvedere College (S.J.) and University College, Dublin, he holds bachelor degrees in both psychology and clinical hypnotherapy and, in 1990, earned his doctorate in Clinical Hypnotherapy. He holds Master Practitioner Certifications in Neuro-Linguistic Programming (NLP), certified by the Society of NLP, and in Time Line Therapy. He is also trained to diagnostics level in Though Field Therapy (Callaghan Techniques). In addition, he holds certification in adjunctive therapies including Mayr Cure and Vega BioKinesiology.

He has completed over ten thousand hours of one-to-one therapy with clients and more than two thousand hours of group work. Together with Rhoda Draper he has been involved in research in the applications of Behavioural Medicine since 1996.

He is a member of the Working Group on the Regulation of Complementary Therapists established by the Minister for Health in Ireland.

Currently, he lectures in clinical applications of Ericksonian hypnosis and Behavioural Medicine and presents courses for patients in these subjects.

RHODA DRAPER was educated in Dublin, at Loreto Convent, Foxrock, Rosslyn House, Weybridge, Surrey, and at Trinity College, Dublin where, as a mature student, she graduated with an honour degree in psychology. She now works as a psychotherapist in private practice in Dublin, specialising in anxiety-related conditions and, together with Dr. Sean Collins, has been involved in research in the applications of Behavioural Medicine since 1996 .

In addition to Master Practitioner certification in Ericksonian Hypnotherapy and Neuro-Linguistic Programming, she is an approved trainer in Thought Field Therapy (Callahan Techniques). She is also a certified TFT Diagnostics Practitioner and has a diploma in Applied Behavioural Medicine.

She currently lectures in Ericksonian Hypnosis, Neuro-Linguistic Programming and Thought Field Therapy™.